PHYLOGENETICS

Edited by **Ibrokhim Y. Abdurakhmonov**

Phylogenetics
http://dx.doi.org/10.5772/63115
Edited by Ibrokhim Y. Abdurakhmonov

Contributors

NiteenV Patil, ChaitanyaG Joshi, Suchitra Sena Dande, Milton Gallardo, Ming Chen, Anatoliy Drozdov, José Luis Fernández-García, Guanghong Zuo, Bailin Hao

Published by InTech

Janeza Trdine 9, 51000 Rijeka, Croatia

Publishing Process Manager Diana Olloni
Technical Editor SPi Global
Cover InTech Design team

First published August, 2017
Printed in Croatia
Legal deposit, Croatia: National and University Library in Zagreb

Additional hard copies can be obtained from orders@intechopen.com

Phylogenetics, Edited by Ibrokhim Y. Abdurakhmonov
p. cm.
Print ISBN 978-953-51-3499-2
Online ISBN 978-953-51-3502-9

For EU product safety concerns:
IN TECH d.o.o., Prolaz Marije Krucifikse Kozulić 3, 51000 Rijeka, Croatia,
info@intechopen.com or visit our website at intechopen.com.

Meet the editor

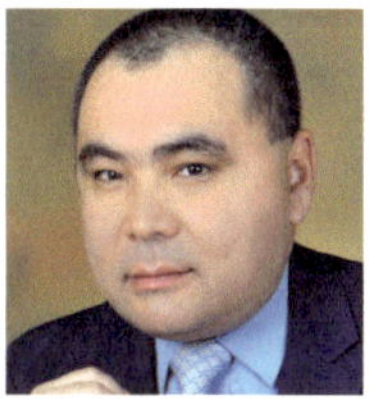

Ibrokhim Y. Abdurakhmonov received his B.S. Degree (1997) in Biotechnology from the National University of Uzbekistan, his M.S. degree in Plant Breeding (2001) from Texas A&M University, USA, his PhD degree (2002) in Molecular Genetics, a Doctor of Science degree (2009) in Genetics, and full professorship (2011) in Molecular Genetics and Molecular Biotechnology from the Institute of Genetics and Plant Experimental Biology, Academy of Sciences of Uzbekistan. He founded (2012) and is currently leading the Center of Genomics and Bioinformatics of Uzbekistan. He serves as an associate editor/editorial board member of several international and national journals on plant sciences. He received several awards including the 2010 Chest Badge "Sign of Uzbekistan" government award, 2010 TWAS prize, and the ICAC Cotton Researcher of the Year 2013- for his outstanding contribution to cotton genomics and biotechnology. He was elected as The World Academy of Sciences (TWAS) Fellow (2014) in Agricultural Science and as a co-chair/chair of the "Comparative genomics and Bioinformatics" workgroup (2015) for the International Cotton Genome Initiative (ICGI). In 2017, he was elected as a Vice President of the Academy of Sciences of Uzbekistan.

Contents

Preface

The word phylogenetics comes from the combination of the Greek words "phylé" or "phylon" meaning tribe or family, and "geneticos" meaning the origin of relatedness; therefore, *Phylogenetics* aims to study the evolutionary relatedness of living organisms on our planet. While addressing and targeting the study of relatedness of living matter on Earth, phylogenetics attempts to evolutionarily connect the origin and spread of living organisms or their populations by applying various mathematical models as well as bioinformatics tools and novel computing techniques. These models reconstruct historical relationships that we cannot see at present and infer evolutionary events and missing chains that help to explain the current 'Tree of Life.' At the same time, phylogenetics allows us to predict the future changes that may happen in the 'Tree of Life,' estimating its rate and future consequences. Therefore, the application of *Phylogenetics* is extended but not limited to evolution, classification and taxonomy of living organisms; ecology, diversity, and conservation biology of agrobiocenosis; forensic analyses; and monitoring of pathogen spread, outbreaks and source of transmissions, useful for novel public health or agricultural biosecurity policies.

Historically, phylogenetics studies were prevalently based on morphological features (phenetics) of species that helped to classify the 'Tree of Life' on Earth. Although still useful for detecting approximate phylogenetic relationships, due to the fact that the same morphological traits could arise independently and be analogous by occurrence, in some specific cases morphology-based phylogenetic conclusions may be misleading and not reliable. Hence, modern phylogenetics studies rely more heavily on molecular sequence data including DNAs, RNAs, proteins, etc. The result of phylogenetics analyses based on both morphology and molecular data is a diagrammatic depiction of relatedness, which is known as a phylogenetic tree. This is the most attractive side of *Phylogenetics* and helps to explain complex knowledge of relatedness, evolution and divergence of life in a simple pictorial level, where topology, rooting, nodding and branching patterns of a tree carry very important information on relatedness estimates that require specific skills to extract needed information with application of appropriate validation tools.

Phylogenetics studies have significantly increased over the past 50 years. The number of scientific publications on phylogenetics have drastically increased and as of June 2017, reached 3,415 scientific publications, indexed in *PubMed* database (https://www.ncbi.nlm.nih.gov/pubmed/?term=phylogenetics), with its first raise in 1995-2000, following a significant increase after 2010. Phylogenetics studies have been more impacted by the recent development genomics and bioinformatics sciences in the genomics and post-genomics era. The emergence and availability of inexpensive, high-throughput next generation sequencing technologies together with the development of computing tools of large-scale biomedical data have shifted phylogenetics studies to new levels that are helping to solve many uncertainty cases in the 'Tree of Life.'

In this *Phylogenetics* book, therefore, we aimed to present readers the latest advances in phylogenetics studies. Toward this goal, we succeeded to compile six chapters with a broad coverage of phylogenetics topics that include multi-kingdom system-based megasystimatics, new phylogenetic approaches for conservation biology, cytogenetics-based comparative phylogeny, phylogenetics of complex polyploidy genomes with reticulated evolution, metagenomics-based phylogenetics of faecal microbiomes of pack animals, and whole genome-based phylogeny tools for prokaryotic organisms.

Although not all classical and modern phylogenetics topics, existing analyses tools and perspective directions are covered by this edited volume, chapters do represent and re-visit some past and current highlights of phylogenetics research, which I believe will be interesting and an additional reading resource for scientists, students and readers of life science direction.

I thank all authors of the book chapters for their valuable contributions. I also thank the InTechOpen book department for giving me the opportunity to work on this book project, and Ms. Diana Olloni, InTechOpen's Publishing Process Manager, for her coordination of this book project.

Ibrokhim Y. Abdurakhmonov
Center of Genomics and Bioinformatics,
Academy of Sciences of Uzbekistan,
Tashkent, Uzbekistan

Dedication

*"In a memory of the First President of Uzbekistan, **Islam Karimov**, and my former advisor at Texas A&M University, Emeritus Professor**Kaml El-Zik** - two great men with my untellable affection and gratitude for supporting my education and inspiring me to believe that I was capable of becoming a scientist ."*

Section 1

Phylogenetic for Taxonomy, Reticulated Evolution and Conservation Biology

Chapter 1

Principle of Conservatism of Cellular Structures as the Basis for Construction of the Multikingdom System of the Organic Word

Anatoliy L. Drozdov

Additional information is available at the end of the chapter

http://dx.doi.org/10.5772/intechopen.68562

Abstract

This chapter describes the history of megasystematics (taxonomy of higher taxons) from Karl Linnaeus till the present day. Nowadays, the Whittaker's five-kingdom system of cellular organisms is the best known. This system has made monophyletic the kingdoms of plants, fungi, and animals but increased the heterogeneity of the kingdom Protoctista. There is one of the qualitative peculiarities of the subcellular level of the organization of living systems, which has been named "the principle of conservatism." We offer the multikingdom system of cellular organisms, based on this principle. In many ways, it can be done based on intuition. We promote the concept of three branches of cellular organisms that is accepted in megasystematics. It is proposed to give these branches of organic word the rank of domains Archaea, Bacteria, and Eucarya. The Empire Cellulata is divided into three domains, which, in turn, are divided into several kingdoms. Our system contains 26 kingdoms.

Keywords: history of megasystematics, multikingdom phylema, the most primitive eukaryotes

1. Introduction

The history of megasystematics (taxonomy of higher taxons) dates back to the eighteenth century when a classification system of the living beings was created by the father of systematics (or taxonomy) Karl Linnaeus, which comprised two kingdoms—Vegetabilia and Animalia

(**Figure 1**). In the nineteenth century, the kingdom of fungi (Mycetoideum), on the one hand, and the kingdom of Protista or Protoctista, on the other, uniting unicellular or most of the lower organisms, were erected; however, most biologists continued adhering to the two-kingdom system.

The system of R.H. Whittaker is the most frequently adopted. He recognizes in his later work [1–4] the prokaryote as a kingdom Monera and divides the eukaryotes into three kingdoms—higher kingdoms of plants, fungi, and animals, which as three stocks were transferred by him from the lower kingdom of Protista (**Figure 2**).

In that classification scheme, red and brown algae were placed near the base of the stock of plants, green algae were placed both in the protist kingdom (apparently, unicellular forms) and at the base of the plant kingdom, whereas myxomycetes were positioned near the base of the stock of fungi. This system is the most popular and in common use till date. The frequently adopted is Whittaker's five-kingdom system of cellular organisms modified by Lynn Margulis [5–8]. She thus made monophyletic the kingdoms of plants, fungi, and animals but increased the heterogeneity of the kingdom Protoctista. L. Margulis herself frankly admitted that "the

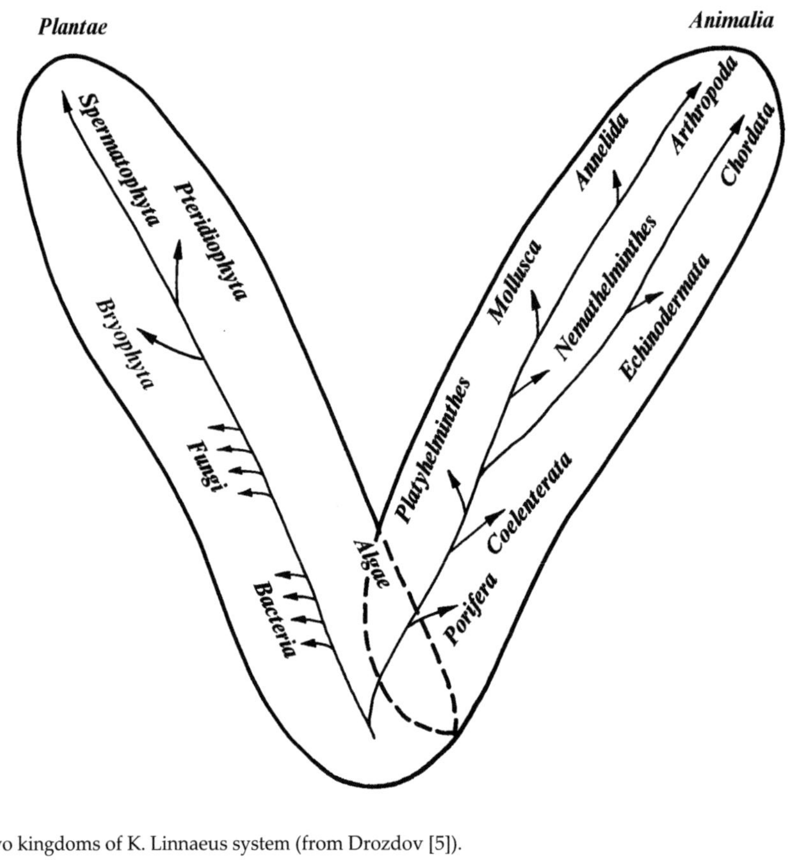

Figure 1. Two kingdoms of K. Linnaeus system (from Drozdov [5]).

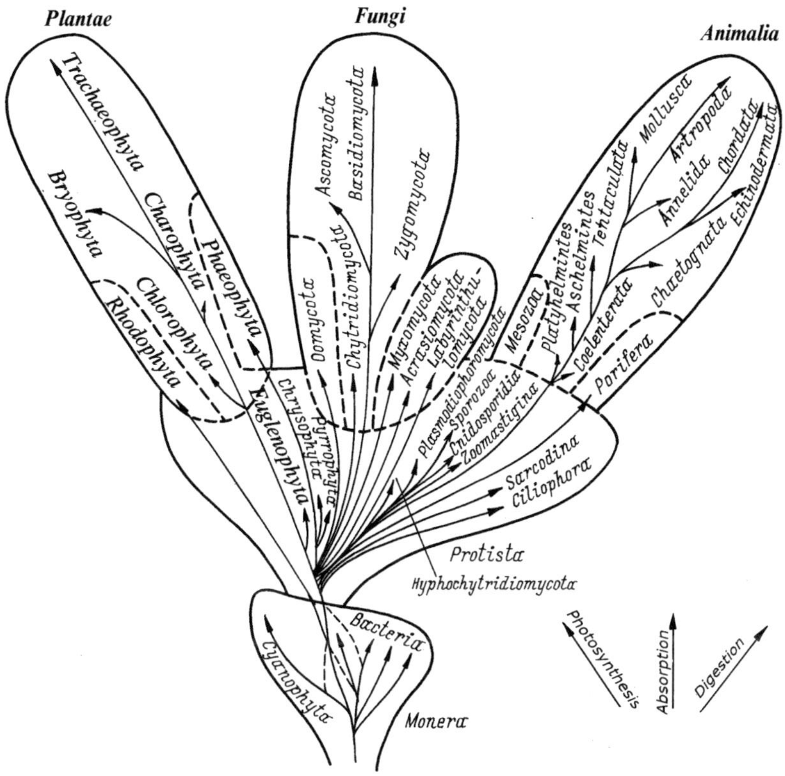

Figure 2. Five kingdoms of R. Whittaker system (from Drozdov [5]).

protoctist kingdom becomes looking as if it were a dump." From these words of L. Margulis, it unambiguously follows that all schemes with few eukaryotic kingdoms (1–4) will err toward inadmissible polyphyly, as is confirmed by contemporary cytological and, especially, molecular biology data.

2. History of megasystematics

Whittaker's scheme was one of the last systems where adaptive features are interwoven with truly phylogenetic characteristics, that is, convergent similarity is claimed to be affinity. Being an ecologist, R.H. Whittaker himself pointed to the adaptive character of evolution of three higher kingdoms, which are connected with their feeding mode: plants are generally autotrophs, fungi feed by absorption, whereas animals are characterized by holozoic nutrition and digestion. R.H. Whittaker indicated this main trend in evolution with three arrows near each of the three higher kingdoms. As regards higher plants (development of the root, conductive system, orifices, reduction of gametophyte, and then loss of flagellate stage, appearance of seed and fruit), true fungi (loss of flagella), and higher vertebrates (appearance of amnion, egg enclosed by membranes, or viviparity), their progressive evolution is not related to feeding, but rather it is connected with adaptation for life on land and with the abandonment of whatever, even temporary, residence in the aquatic environment. It is no occasion that both the botanist Zernov [9] and the ecologist Odum [10, 11] considered Whittaker's scheme to be a functional, i.e. (*id est*), ecological, rather than a taxonomic one, and Y. Odum emphasized that his kingdoms, which are "functional kingdoms," should not be confused with taxonomic ones, although there are some parallels. It is therefore natural that L. Margulis, when revising Whittaker's system, replaced these arrows with another ones, indicating haplo-diploid nature of plants, diploid nature of animals, dikaryoid nature of fungi, and haploid nature of algae.

Other systems have been considered by us in details [12, 13]. In them [14–19], the eukaryotes are subdivided into 6–18 kingdoms. Thus, Edwards [16] proposed to distribute plants among seven kingdoms belonging to two subkingdoms of Prokaryota (kingdom of blue-green algae) and eukaryotic plants with six kingdoms: Erythrobionta with one division Rhodophyta, Chlorobionta embracing four divisions (Chlorophyta, Bryophyta, Tracheophyta, and Euglenophyta), Ochrobionta comprising four divisions (Phaeophyta, Chrysophyta, Cryptophyta, and Pyrrophyta), Myxobionta with four divisions (Myxogastriomycota, Dictyosteliomycota, Acrasiomycota, and Protosteliomycota), Fungi 1 with four divisions (Zygomycota, Ascomycota, Basidiomycota, and Chytridiomycota), and Fungi 2 comprising three divisions (Labyrinthulomycota, Hyphochytridiomycota, and Oomycota). One can concur with most of Edwards' kingdoms. Division of fungi into two kingdoms is well-grounded. All divisions of Fungi 2 are now assigned to the same kingdom as Ochrobionta. Only Myxobionta are now removed from plants and distributed among two kingdoms.

After K. Linnaeus, the author of system, as well as J. Cuvie, who introduced the high-rank category of phylum, which also proved very useful, was the first case. The category of domain was set forth later.

It has become absolutely clear that the major high-rank taxonomic categories of Linnaeus are insufficient and new ones are needed. The simplest way is using additional categories such as subphylum, subkingdom, and superkingdom. Many scientists went this way, but, in doing so, they were compelled to introduce more categories such as "Uberreich," "Oberreich," "Unterreic" [19] or "Superkingdom," "Subphylum," "Infraphylum," and "Parvikingdom" [20–24].

Vorontsov [26–28] was the first who introduced into scientific usage a major taxonomic category higher in rank than kingdom, the empire. He recognized two empires: of precellular organisms in which he placed a single kingdom, that of viruses, and the empire of cellular organisms embracing two subempires: subempire of prenucleate organisms comprising bacteria and blue-green algae and the subempire of nucleate organisms (or eukaryotes). The introduction of such high-level taxonomic category as the empire is of much importance for taxonomy and quite a bold suggestion.

3. Principle of conservatism of subcellular structures

The multikingdom system of the organic world was advanced by us [11, 12, 28–30]. It was based on the principle of conservatism of cellular structures formulated by Mashansky and Drozdov [31, 32]. There is a biological paradox: the subcellular structures are highly conservative.

While discussing the structural foundations of biological systems, we should not limit our attention by fixing it only to the correlation of various levels of the organization of living matter, to what we are used to call the problem of integration. We have to realize that every single level is unique in its qualitative specificity and particular features.

There is an enormous variety of cells. They differ in their morphology, functions, and their chemical structure. However, when we proceed to the next, the so-called subcellular level, we are confronted with the fact that the principal structure of basic cellular organelles, such as membranes, mitochondria, centrioles, filaments, ribosomes, endoplasmatic reticulum, and Golgi apparatus, remains unchanged in a wide variety of objects. In the hierarchical sequence of the organizational levels of biological systems, it is the subcellular level, and that merits ever greater attention for its most remarkable characteristic feature, namely its membranous structure—its supermolecular system of proteins, lipids, and polysaccharides of several types. We can be certain to expect some new properties to be discovered typical of the structure and functions of cellular organelles on account of the peculiarities of their level of organization.

There are only two variants of the ultrastructure of biological membranes (lipid bilayer in Eubacteria and Eukaryotes and single layer in Archaebacteria), two variants of ribosomes, six variants of ultrastructural organization of plastids, three variants of organization of mitochondria, three variants of organization of nuclear apparatus, and three variants of organization of kinetic apparatus.

A suitable object for a comparative morphological analysis is presented by mitochondria. For identifying of mitochondria can be taken the typical organization of their membranes. The lipoprotein nature of mitochondrial membranes does not cause any doubt, neither does the similarity of these membranes to the ones belonging to other organelles. Yet, there are data on the mitochondrial membrane testifying to its structural as well as functional uniqueness.

Mitochondria are remarkable for the great variety of their organizations. There are lamellar or tubular crysts that can exist singly or densely packed, or they can be either scattered or highly organized. There can be several small mitochondria in a cell, or a single one spreading over a large number of shoots: there can be one mitochondrion in a cell, or quite a number of them densely packed together. Despite such great variety, the general pattern of the structure of mitochondria invariably repeats itself—it is one and the same in mushrooms, algae, multicellular animals, and plants. There are four types of structures of the crysts of mitochondria—the lamellar, the tubular, the tubularly vesicular, and discoid one. The nature of mechanisms determining the morphology of mitochondrial crysts is unknown yet. Nevertheless, the functional peculiarities of the cells are of considerable significance. Thus, in the cells synthesizing steroid hormones, we find mitochondria with tubularly vesicular crysts. However, an injection of steroid hormones to lower invertebrate allows to transform the mitochondria of the neurons with typically lamellar crysts into those with tubularly vesicular ones [31].

Mitochondria can cardinally change their ultrastructure under the impact of alternating factors or training. This signifies high liability in mitochondria, the ultrastructure of which is determined by the function of the cells irrespective of the systematic position of the object. On the basis of presently available material on the ultrastructure of mitochondria of the cells of a great variety of tissues as well as the specificity of their responses to various alternating factors, it is possible to state that there are no convincing facts which might permit to fix any correlations between the level of phylogenetic position, or ontogeny and the ultrastructure of mitochondria in investigated species belonging to different realms of living organisms. All the observed differences in the ultrastructure of mitochondria can be accounted for by their functional peculiarities, their loads during a certain period of activity. There, evidently, lies one of the qualitative peculiarities of the subcellular level of the organization of living systems, which has been named "the principle of conservatism" [31, 32].

These facts demonstrating the lack of changes in cellular organelles, such as rather intricate in their organization mitochondria, during the long process of their evolution give a reason to conclude that already at the early stages of evolution, the structural as well as chemical organization of living systems was rather complicated and well developed. This fact calls for a discussion of the problems of the early stages of evolution, beginning with the appearance of life on Earth, which is currently widely discussed on various levels, and extreme views are being stated.

The uniformity of the structure of cellular organelles, such as mitochondria and, perhaps, even those of a more intricate organization, namely filaments, gives grounds to view them as structures formed on one single occasion. The structure of nucleic acids has a common origin in all living systems. This conclusion is prompted by the widely known uniformity of the code formed on four bases.

The above-mentioned conception should explain why mitochondria have a genetic code that differs very slightly from that of the nucleus as well as that of the prokaryotes. In fact, the code of mitochondria differs very little from the universal one. Only five codons have different meaning: methionine, isoleucine, tryptophan, and, also, a changed terminator. While analyzing these divergences, it is possible to see that the code of mitochondria is nearer to the quasidouble "ideal" one. This may testify the fact that the code of mitochondria is more ancient than the universal one. Possibly, there was a time when all cells had a code similar to that of present-day mitochondria. Then, some changes occurred in the general code, but in mitochondria, the code proved to be more stable. The reason for this may lie in the small size of the genome of mitochondria and so every mutation brought about such changes in the characteristics that proved lethal.

There is another important problem, namely, why the mitochondrial genetic system, once formed, survived in the evolution practically unchanged, and how could it preserve its independence in the cell. Mahler and coauthors [33] suggested the opinion that, as polypeptides coded by DNA and belonging to mitochondrial complexes are rather hydrophobic, they must be synthesized somewhere near the place of their inclusion into the mitochondrial membrane and cannot be transported through the cell. Probably, the preservation of mt-DNA throughout the evolution was due to it serving as a supplier of the functionally indispensable elements to mitochondria.

We believe that the most topical, fruitful, and perspective objective of megasystematics is the elaboration of multikingdom system consisting of monophyletic taxa, and we are aware of all difficulties of this task. One of the main difficulties is that now in a boiling cauldron of new information, one can hardly make a whatever stable system. There are many reasons for this. The ultrastructure of many protists has not yet been studied; the structure of many organisms is either very peculiar or unclear so that they cannot be classified with the existing taxa of even high rank; the degree of conservatism of cellular structures is being elucidated; and the techniques for demonstrating relatedness are being improved. It is, therefore, no accident that different authors recognize different number of kingdoms, and the authors themselves sometimes remake their systems too hastily. Thus, Cavalier-Smith [34] delineates seven kingdoms among the eukaryotes; 3 years later, he already recognized nine kingdoms, and later he reduced the number of kingdoms to six [21–24, 35–39].

4. Multikingdom systems of the organic world

Nevertheless, the adherents of monophyletic system have made tremendous progress. The kingdom Ochrobiontes (Chromobionta or Chromista) is distinctly delineated; along with a number of divisions of chlorophyll *C*-containing algae, it embraces some groups from the kingdoms Fungi and Protozoa. The kingdom Viridiplantae comprises all green algae Chlorophyta s. lato, bryophytes, and higher plants but no more; the kingdom Metazoa (but not Animalia!) is also monophyletic. Some kingdoms are not as clearly delineated as Euglenobiontes, Alveolates, Cryptobiontes, Prymnesiobiontes, etc. are. However, some groups, among them Foraminifera, Radiolaria s. lato, and others, have not yet been placed properly. Instead of being squeezed, without due grounds, into the existing kingdoms, these groups should rather be regarded as groups incertae sedis, as is done by many taxonomists.

When analyzing the old system, in which features of adaptive similarity and phylogenetic relatedness turned out to be intermingled, there is an increasing criticism from various investigators that many taxa are not monophyletic but rather ecomorphological notions. Shafranova [40] addressed this problem in her paper "Plant as a Life Form." Mirabdullaev [41, 42] correctly points out that the former system of protists was primarily the system of life forms (ecomorphs) rather than phylogenetic taxa and that similar structural patterns can arise convergently. Many foreign scientists are now coming to analogous conclusions. Here, the question arises: what should be done with out-dated, traditional notions that serve no longer as taxa, namely plants, protists, animals, heliozoans, flagellates, sporozoans, etc. To avoid extremely troublesome and even unnecessary rejection of old terminology, many researchers began using them not as taxa but as designations of ecomorphs or life forms [43, 44]. This does not necessarily imply that the existing terminology should be changed radically. Up to now, in botanical institutions, mycologists have successfully worked hand in hand with algologists, and both prokaryotic bacteria and eukaryotic fungi have been applied in microbiological industry.

Moreover, it has turned out that these terms can and must be used in the ecomorphological system or the system of life forms, which has long been a necessity. Teofrast's system was one of early attempts at constructing such a system. To date, a variety of such systems have been created at different levels. Unfortunately, the ecomorphological system was elaborated independently of the taxonomic one, which was thought of as if being something stable, and its terms were little used. The adoption and use of the terms that are well established in taxonomy were not appropriate for the new system. Thus, in his ecomorphological system, which is one of the better developed, for high-rank taxa, he retains the names "Kingdom," "Division," "Phylum," and "Class," which can cause only confusion. Barr's viewpoint seems to be more correct [44]. Only for fungi, he proposed two systems: a phylogenetic one, where fungi were distributed among three kingdoms—Eumycota, Chromista, and Protozoa—and an ecological one, in which fungi in the old sense constitute union 1 of Fungi.

The idea is to create, on the basis of the old system in which the genetic and ecomorphological criteria were intermingled, two parallel systems—the phylema or phylogenetic, taxonomic system and the ecomorphological system. The elaboration of the ecomorphological system is a very complicated task, although much has been done in this respect. Without doubt, many descriptive terms of traditional systematics will find their place in the new system.

At present a lot of biologists study the problems of megasystematics. Close with our megasystem was build up the system by Leontiev and Akulov [45]. But most of new systems limit themselves to study the sequence of nucleotide in ribosomal RNA. The molecular biologists studying rRNA work at different countries—in USA, Canada, Belgium, Japan, and different European countries like Russia. There are a few sites in Internet, where the phylogenetic trees are represented. A lot of such trees were published last years. Attention should be paid to the discussion of their systems as variant of five-kingdom system. Nevertheless, Cavalier-Smith [20–24, 34–39] already published the six to nine kingdoms systems. He comprises two empires—Prokaryota and Eukaryota.

Since the end of year 1970, the concept of three branches of cellular organisms is accepted in megasystematics [46]. It is proposed to give these branches of organic word the rank of domains Archaea, Bacteria, and Eucarya [47–51]. Therefore, the empire Cellulata is divided to three domains, which, in turn, are divided into several kingdoms [25, 39] (**Figures 3–7**).

The scheme reflects the great diversity of life forms of bacteria adapted to living in almost all ecological niches. Some of them such as *Ancalochloris* (1), *Aquaspirillum* (2), and *Chromatin* (3) live in water, whereas *Aquaspirillum* can use a chain of magnetized particles to find sediments, rich in nutrient agents. *Haloarcula* (4) are distributed in the saline marshes. *Pyrodictium* (5) prefers hot places; *Rhizobium* (6) settles in the roots of plants and produces nitrogen available to the host tissue form. Type of bacteria: *Escherichia* (7), *Streptococcus* (8),

http://dx.doi.org/10.5772/intechopen.68562

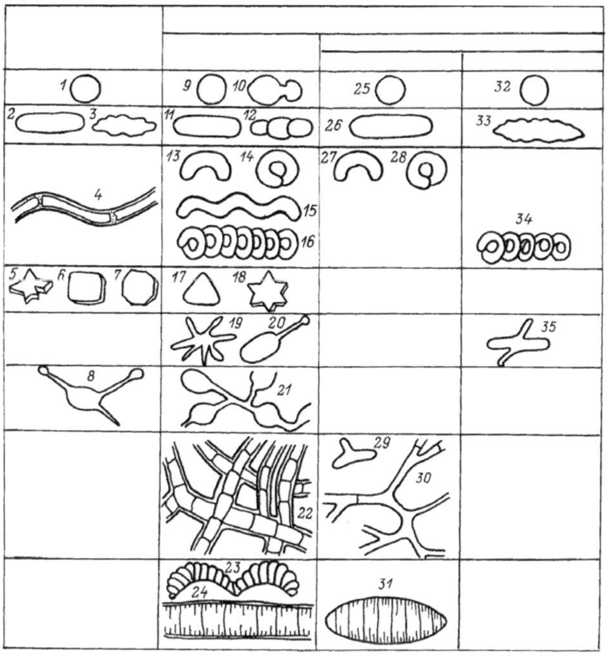

Figure 3. The main bacteria morphotypes (from Kussakin, Drozdov [11]). Archaebacteria: 1, *Methanococcus;* 2, *Methanobacterium, Halobacterium;* 3, *Thermoplasma;* 4, *Methanospirillum;* 5, *Haloarcula;* 6, square bacteria; 7, *Sulfolobus;* 8, *Pyrodictium.* Gram-negative bacteria (Gracilicutes): 9, *Neisseria, Veillonella;* 10, *Gemmiger;* 11, *Escherichia;* 12, *Seliberia;* 13, *Vibrio, Bdellovibrio;* 14, *Mycrocyclus;* 15, *Spirillum;* 16, *Spirochaeta;* 17, *Angulomicrobium;* 18, *Stella;* 19, *Prosthecomicrobium;* 20, *Caulobacter;* 21, *Hyphomicrobium, Rhodomicrobium;* 22, *Mastigocoleus;* 23, *Simonsiella;* 24, *Oscillochloris, Oscillatoria.* Gram-positive bacteria (Firmicutes): 25, *Micrococcus;* 26, *Bacillus, Erysipelothrix;* 27 and 28, *Desulfotomaculum, Clostridium;* 29, *Mycobacterium;* 30, *Streptomyces;* 31, *Caryophanon, Oscillospira.* Mycoplasma (Tenericutes): 32, 33, and 35, *Mycoplasma;* 34, *Spiroplasma.*

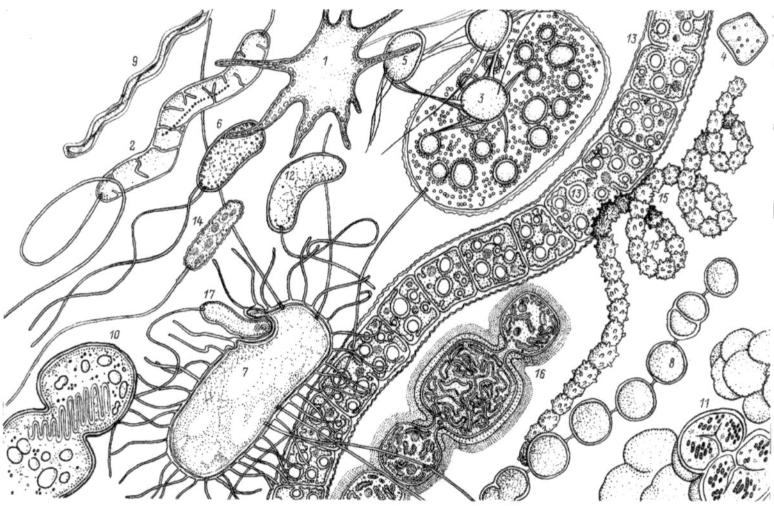

Figure 4. The different forms of Eubacteria (from Drozdov [5]).

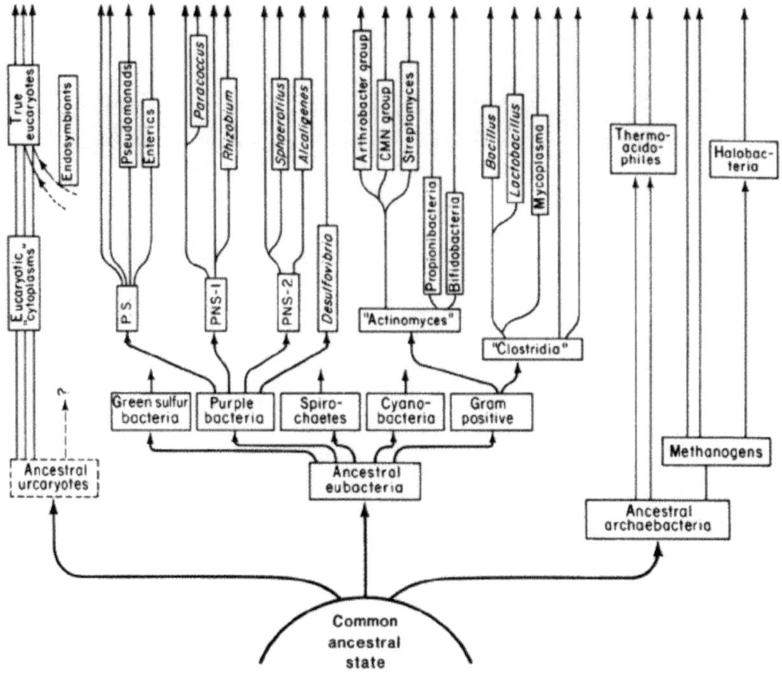

Figure 5. Schematic representation of the major lines of prokaryotic descent (after Fox et al. [46]).

and *Treponema* (9) cause various diseases in humans. The metabolism requirements can combine incompatible species of bacteria: aerobic methane consumer *Methylococcus* (10)

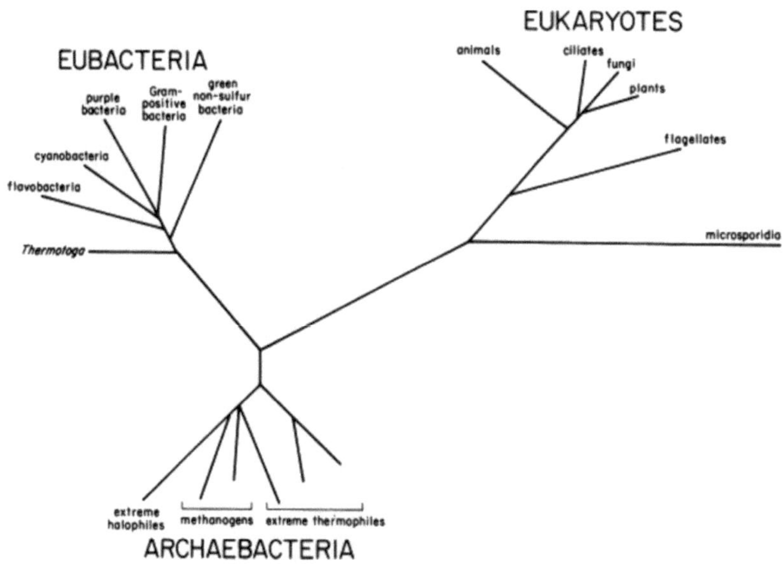

Figure 6. Unrooted tree shows the three branch of organic word (after Woese [49]).

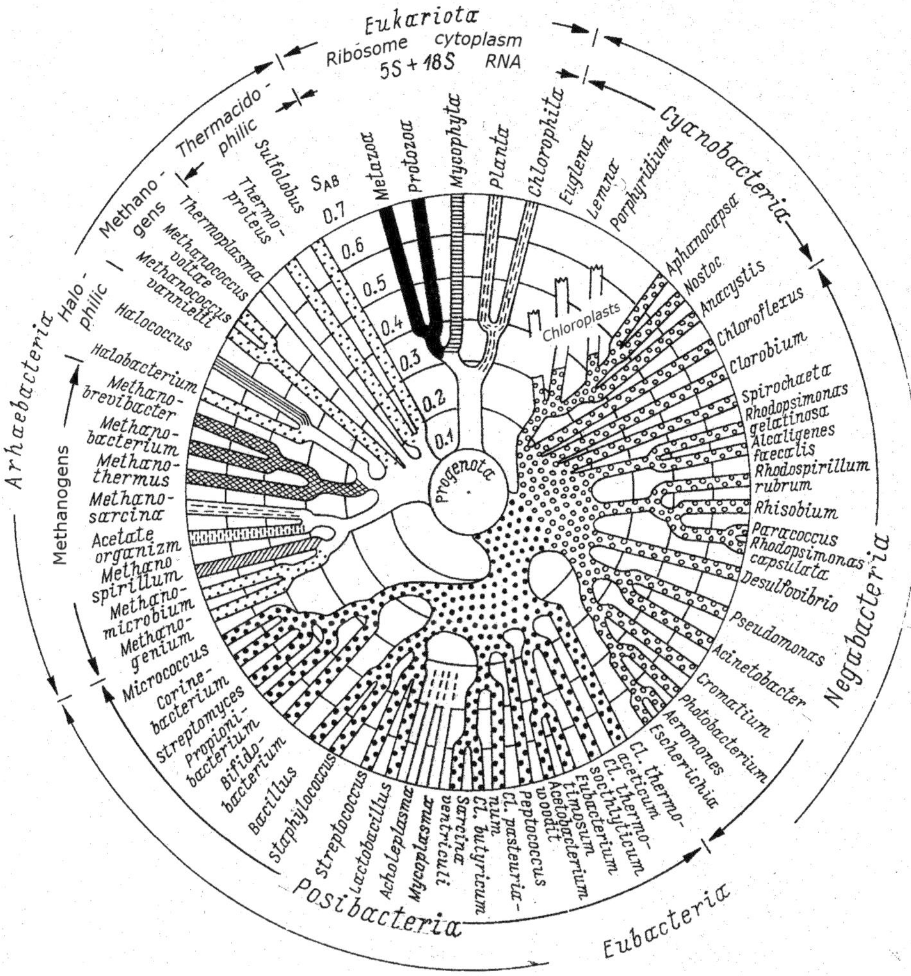

Figure 7. Kandler ring. The phylogenetic unrooted tree constructed on base of analysis rRNA and cell wall (for prokaryotes) (after Kandler [52]).

draws *Methanosarcina* (11), and anaerobic producing methane *Desulfovibrio* (12), producing hydrogen sulfide—*Ancalochloris* (1), *Beggitoa* (13), and *Chromatium* (3)— requires hydrogen sulfide. Another group of bacteria, consuming hydrogen sulfide, *Thiobacillus* (14), is used for extraction of metals from ore. *Streptomyces* (15) secrete antibiotics. *Anabaena* (16) produces oxygen from water in the process of photosynthesis, whereas *Bdellovibrio* attacks many other bacteria (17).

We support this idea and propose to distinguish 4 kingdoms in Archaebacteria, 7 kingdoms in Eubacteria, and 15 kingdoms in Eukaryotes. Our system we represent as scheme (**Figure 8**) and as the table (**Table 2**). In **Table 1**, we propose the next ends for word of designations of taxa on levels kingdom, phylum, class and order.

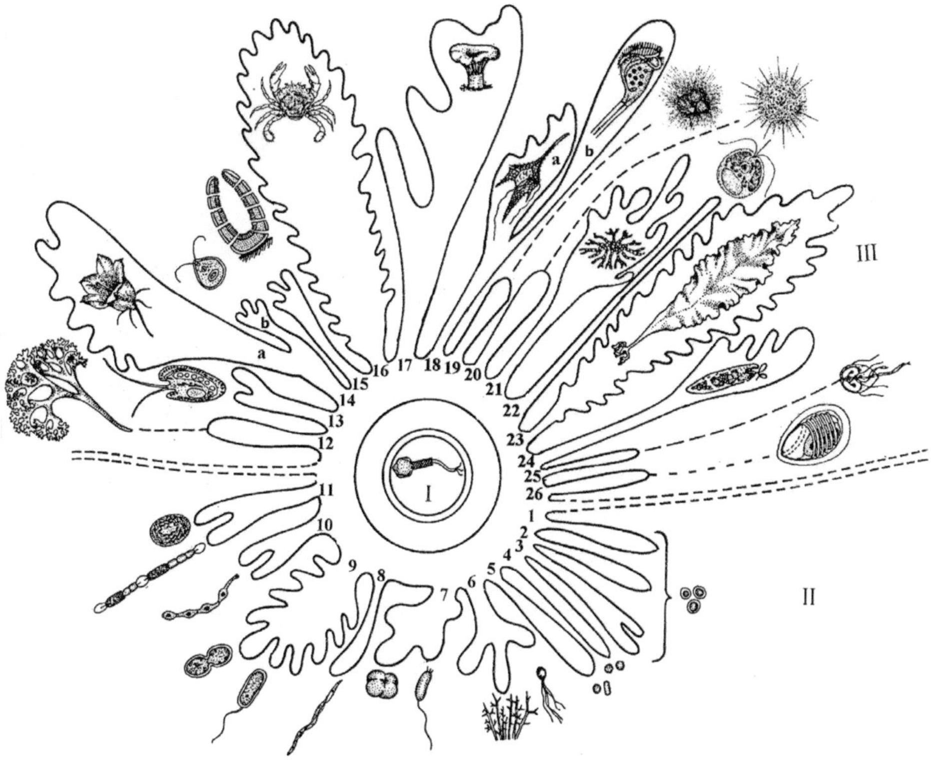

Figure 8. The multikingdom phylogenetic unrooted tree constructed on base of principle of conservatism (after Drozdov [5]). I, Virae; II, Prokaryotes: 1, Methanobacteriobiontes; 2, Halobacteriobiontes; 3, Thermoacidobacteriobiontes; 4, Archaetenericutobacteriobiontes; 5, Tenericotobacteriobiontes; 6, Actinobacteriobiontes; 7, Firmicutobacteriobiontes; 8, Spirochaetobacteriobiontes; 9, Scotobacteriobiontes; 10, Anoxyphotobacteriobiontes; 11, Oxyphotobacteriobiontes; III, Eukaryotes: 12, Rhodobiontes; 13, Cryptobiontes; 14, Chlorobiontes (a, Thallobionti; б, Embryobionti); 15, Parazoobiontes; 16, Metazoobiontes; 17, Mycobiontes; 18, Alveolatobiontes (a, Peridiniobionti; b, Parameciobionti); 19, Foraminiferobiontes; 20, Radiolariobiontes; 21, Myxobiontes; 22, Prymnesiobiontes; 23, Heterokontobiontes; 24, Euglenobiontes; 25, Archaemonadobiontes; 26, Microsporobiontes.

Category	Applicable ends	Category	Applicable ends
Superkingdom	-obiontoi	Superclassis	-idees
Kingdom	-obiontes	Classis	--indes
Subkingdom	-obiontoi	Subclassis	-iones
Superphylum	-ophylaces	Superorder	-iformi
Phylum	-ophylea	Order	-iformes
Subphylum	-ophylinea	Suborder	-oidei

Table 1. Applicable ends for word of designations of taxa on kingdom, phylum, classis, and order taxonomic rank.

http://dx.doi.org/10.5772/intechopen.68562

Imperia Cellulata

Dominion Archaebacteria

I. Kingdom Thermoacidobacteriobiontes

1. Phylum Sulfolobophyles

2. Phylum Thermoproteophyles

II. Kingdom Archaetenericutobacteriobiontes

3. Phylum Thermoplasmophyles

III. Kingdom Halobacteriobiontes

4. Phylum Halobacteriophyles

5. Phylum Halococcophyles

IV. Kingdom Methanobacteriobiontes

6. Phylum Methanobacteriophyles

Dominion Eubacteria

Superkingdom Gracilicutobiontoi

V. Kingdom Cyanobiontes (Oxyphotobacteriobiontes)

7. Phylum Nostocophyles

8. Phylum Prochlorophyles

VI. Kingdom Anoxyphotobacteriobiontes

9. Phylum Rhodospirillophyles

10. Phylum Chlorobiophyles

VII. Kingdom Scotobacteriobiontes

11. Phylum Thiobacillophyles

12. Phylum Desulfovibriophyles

13. Phylum Azotobacteriophyles

14. Phylum Pseudomonadophyles

15. Phylum Enterobacteriophyles

16. Phylum Bacteroidophyles

17. Phylum Caulobacteriophyles

18. Phylum Myxobacteriophyles

19. Phylum Cytophagophyles

20. Phylum Ricketsiophyles

21. Phylum Chlamydiophyles

VIII. Kingdom Spirochaetobacteriobiontes

22. Phylum Spirochaetophyles

Superkingdom Firmicutobiontoi

IX. Kingdom Actinobacteriobiontes

23. Phylum Mycobacteriophyles

24. Phylum Corynebacteriophyles

25. Phylum Actinomycetophyles

X. Kingdom Eufirmicutobiontes

26. Phylum Clostridiophyles

27. Phylum Bacillophyles

28. Phylum Lactobacillophyles

29. Phylum Micrococcophyles

XI. Kingdom Tenericutobiontes

30. Phylum Mycoplasmophyles

Dominion Eukaryota

XII. Kingdom Microsporobiontes

31. Phylum Microsporidiophyles

XIII. Kingdom Archemonadobiontes

Superphylum Archamoebophylacei

32. Phylum Pelomyxophyles

Class Pelornyxiodes

Class Mastigamoeboides

Superphylum Metamonadophylacei

33. Phylum Retortomonadophyles

34. Phylum Hexamitophyles

35. Phylum Oxymonadophyles

Superphylum Parabasaliophylacei

36. Phylum Trichomonadophyles

Class Trichonymphiodes

XIV. Kingdom Euglenobiontes

Subkingdom Percolobionti

37. Phylum Acrasiophyles

Class Vahlkampfiiodes

Class Acrasilodes

http://dx.doi.org/10.5772/intechopen.68562

Class Percolomonadiodes

Class Lyromonadioides

Subkingdom Euglenobionti

38. Phylum Stephanopogonophyles

39. Phylum Diplonemophyles

40. Phylum Bodonophyles

41. Phylum Euglenophyles

XV. Kingdom Myxobiontes

Subkingdom Myxomycetobionti

42. Phylum Cercomonadophyles

43. Phylum Dictyosteliophyles

44. Phylum Physarophyles

Subkingdom Myxozoobionti

45. Phylum Entamoebophyles

46. Phylum Haplosporophyles

47. Phylum Pararnyxiophyles

48. Phylum Myxidiophyles

XVI. Kingdom Rhodobiontes

49. Phylum Bangiophyles

XVII. Kingdom Alveolatobiontes

Subkingdom Peridiniobionti

Superphylum Peridiniophylacei

50. Phylum Peridiniophyles

Superphylum Apicomplexophylacei

51. Phylum Perkinsophyles

Class Colpodelliodes

Class Perkinsiodes

52. Phylum Gregarinophyles

Subkingdom Parameciobionti

53. Phylum Hemimastigophyles

54. Phylum Parameciophyles

XVIII. Kingdom Heterokontobiontes

55. Phylum Bicosoecophyles

56. Phylum Labyrinthulophyles

57. Phylum Saprolegniophyles

58. Phylum Hyphochytriophyles

59. Phylum Diatomophyles

60. Phylum Triboneroatophyles

61. Phylum Fucophyles

62. Phylum Eustigmatophyles

63. Phylum Synurophyles

64. Phylum Chrysococcophyles

65. Phylum Raphidomonadophyles

66. Phylum Dictyochophyles

67. Phylum Pedinellophyles

Class Pedinelliodes

Class Actinophryiodes

Class Clathruliniodes

Addition to Kingdom Heterokontobiontes

Class Pelagomonadiodes

XIX. Kingdom Foraminiferobiontes

68. Phylum Psamminidophyles (=Xenophyophora)

69. Phylum Foraminiferophyles

70. Phylum Plasmodiophoreophyles

XX. Kingdom Radiolariobiontes

71. Phylum Sphaerozoiophyles (=Polycystinea)

72. Phylum Phaeodiniophyles

73. Phylum Acanthometriophyles

74. Phylum Sticholoncheiophyles

XXI. Kingdom Prymnesiobiontes (=Haptophyta)

75. Phylum Prymnesiophyles (=Haptophyles)

XXII. Kingdom Cryptobiontes

76. Тип Cryptomonadophyles (Cryptophycota)

77. Тип Centrochelidophyles (Acantocystidae)

XXIII. Kingdom Chlorobiontes (=Viridiplantae)

Subkingdom Thallobionti

78. Phylum (Division) Prasinophyles

79. Phylum (Division) Chlorophyles

80. Phylum (Division) Charophyles

Subkingdom Embryobionti (= Cormobionti)

81. Phylum (Division) Bryophyles

82. Phylum (Division) Rhyniophyles (= Psilophyles)

83. Phylum (Division) Psilotophyles

84. Phylum (Division) Lycopodiophyles

85. Phylum (Division) Equisetophyles (Sphenophyles)

86. Phylum (Division) Polypodiophyles (= Filicophyles)

87. Phylum (Division) Pinophyles (= Gymnospermae)

88. Phylum (Division) Magnoliophyles (= Angiospermae)

XXIV. Kingdom Mycobiontes (= Fungi)

Subkingdom Opistomastigomycotobionti

89. Phylum (Division) Chytridiomycotophyles

Subkingdom Amastigomycotobionti (= Eufungi=Eumycota)

90. Phylum (Division) Mucoromycotaphyles (= Zygomycota)

91. Phylum (Division) Trichomycotaphyles

92. Phylum (Division) Ascomycotaphyles

93. Phylum (Division) Basidiomycotaphyles

XXV. Kingdom Parazoobiontes

94. Phylum Choanoflagellata (= Crasperomonadia)

95. Phylum Spongia (= Porifera)

XXVI. Kingdom Metazoobiontes

96. Phylum Placozoa

97. Phylum Cnidaria

98. Phylum Ctenophora

99. Phylum Platyhelminthes

100. Phylum Orthonectida

101. Phylum Nemertini

102. Phylum Entoprocta (= Kamptozoa)

103. Phylum Sipuncula

104. Phylum Mollusca

105. Phylum Echiurida

106. Phylum Annelida

107. Phylum Pogonophora

108. Phylum Vestimentifera
109. Phylum Tardigrada
110. Phylum Pentastomida
111. Phylum Onichophora
112. Phylum Arthropoda
113. Phylum Rotifera
114. Phylum Cycliophora
115. Phylum Acanthocephala
116. Phylum Dicyemataria (= Rhombozoa)
117. Phylum Nemathelminthes
118. Phylum Loricifera
119. Phylum Gastrotricha
120. Phylum Nematomorpha
121. Phylum Priapulida
122. Phylum Kinorhyncha
123. Phylum Chaetognatha
124. Phylum Phoronida
125. Phylum Bryozoa
126. Phylum Brachiopoda
127. Phylum Hemichordata
128. Phylum Echinodermata
129. Phylum Chordata

Incertae sedis: Genera *Gyromitus*; Genera *Discocelis*; Genera *Jacoba*.

Table 2. Multikingdom system of the cellular living beings.

5. The root phylogenetic tree

The construction of a root phylogenetic tree based on the principle of conservatism is not simple. It is necessary to analyze the structure of the six systems of cellular organelles in each Protista group: surface apparatus (membranome), genetic apparatus (karyome), synthetic apparatus (syndetome), mitochondria, plastids, and kinetic apparatus (kinetome). In many ways, it can be done based on intuition. Of course, now the study of the building of phylema of the organic world focuses mainly on the genomic level. Nevertheless, we tried to present phylema of the organic world in a tree, where the kingdom is placed as the complexity of the systems of cellular organelles (**Figure 8**). The main complication is the allocation of the core group in the structure of the tree. It may seem that the problem is simple—the most primitive group includes cells of the simplest arrangement structure. Certainly, the simplest organisms are Microsporobiontes—eukaryotic unicellular intracellular parasites. They have only plasmatic membrane, nucleus, and ribosome. Moreover, their ribosome is closer to 70S-prokaryotic ribosome than to 80S-eukaryotic ribosome. The first molecular studies of ribosomal RNA sequence suggest that Microsporidia are extremely ancient eukaryotes [35, 53]. Later, biochemists discovered that phylogenomics supports Microsporidia as the earliest diverging clade of sequenced fungi [54–59]. Therefore, Microsporidia are secondarily simplified, during adaptation to intracellular anaerobic existence.

The second candidate for the most primitive Eukaryota is the Kingdom Archemonadobiontes with Pelomyxophyles, Retortomonadophyles, Hexamitophyles, Oxymonadophyles, and Trichomonadophyles. They are anaerobic organisms without mitochondria but have from two to numerous flagella. The problem is: had they originally no primary mitochondria or they lost them during adaptation to anaerobic environment? Most professionals concerned with megasystematics are inclined to consider anaerobic eukaryotes as the result of their secondary simplification: they have lost their mitochondria, adapting to obligate anaerobic metabolism.

Rhodobiontes (red algae) had no flagella originally or they have lost them? This is a problem, because they are marine algae only and flagella are necessary organelles in water environment.

6. Conclusion

Euglenoids that have all organelles (membrane with special cell wall, nucleus, 80S ribosome, mitochondria with discoid crista, plastids, and flagella), may be considered as most primitive Eukaryota. According to our system [12], Kingdom Euglenobiontes Leedale, 1974 (from the Greek eu -, in English "good," in compound words it means "well-developed," "authentic," consistent with the ideal and glene—the pupil of the eye) combines the heterotrophic or autotrophic green, usually unicellular monad often amoeboid, but usually with a monadic form in the cycle, rarely colonial organisms. They have and mitochondria with cristae that are usually flattened, rounded with a tapered base—discoid, rarely vesicular, or even less often ribbon-like tube; usually single-nucleus; mitosis in a closed intranuclear ortomitosis; reproduction by a longitudinal division; sexual process is unknown. This kingdom includes two subkingdoms: Euglenobionti and Percolobionti. Although acrasia and heterolobosea amoebas are combined into one common taxon usually called Heterolobosea, we prefer to give it the name from the type genus Acrasia-Acrasiophyles.

With this assumption, understanding of phylogenetics of Eukaryota has no problem. Eukaryota are divided into two branches: Tubulicristata (with mitochondria with tubular crista) and Lamellicristata (with mitochondria with lamellar crista). Cryptomonads occupy an intermediate position with riblike crista and nukleomorf in plastids (**Figure 9** and **Table 2**).

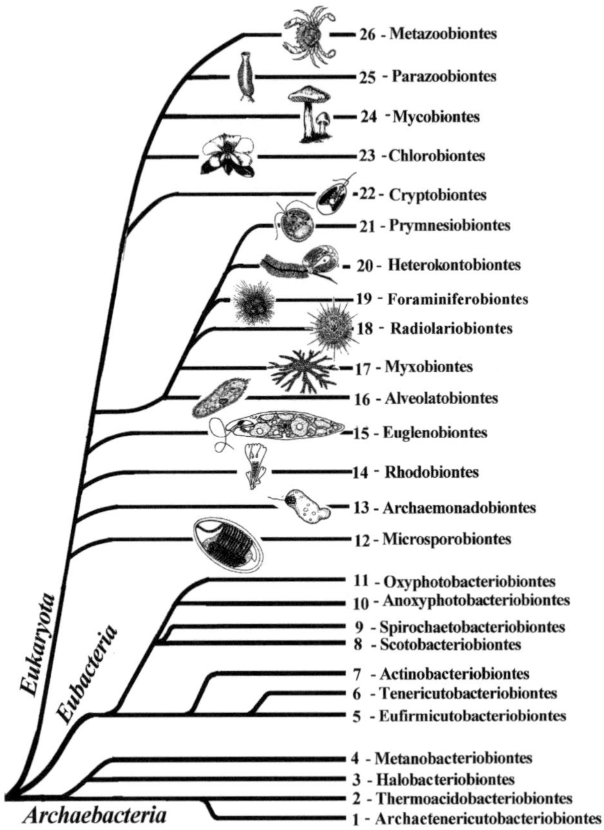

Figure 9. The multikingdom phylogenetic hierarchical tree constructed on base of principle of conservatism (after Drozdov [5]).

Author details

Anatoliy L. Drozdov

*Address all correspondence to: anatoliyld@mail.ru

1 National Scientific Center of Marine Biology, Far Eastern Branch, Russian Academy of Sciences, A.V. Zhirmunsky Institute of Marine Biology FEB RAS, Vladivostok, Russia

2 Far Eastern Federal University, Vladivostok, Russia

References

[1] Whittaker RH. On the broad classification of organisms. The Quarterly Review of Biology. 1959;**34**:210-226

[2] Whittaker RH. New concept of Kingdoms of organisms. Science. 1969;**163**:150-160. Available from: http://www.ib.usp.br/inter/0410113/downloads/Whittaker_1969.pdf

[3] Whittaker RH. Broad classification: The Kingdoms and the protozoans. In: Kreier JP, editor. Parasite Protozoa. Vol. 1. New York and London: Acad. Press; 1977. pp. 1-34

[4] Whittaker RH, Margulis L. Protist classification and the Kingdoms of organisms. BioSystems. 1978;**10**:3-18. Available from: https://www.ncbi.nlm.nih.gov/pubmed/418827

[5] Drozdov AL. Biology for Physicists and Chemists. Vladivostok: Publishing House of Far Eastern State University; 2005. p. 414 (in Russian). Available from: http://search.rsl.ru/ru/record/01003014388

[6] Margulis L. Five-kingdom classification and the origin and evolution of cells. Journal of Evolutionary Biology. 1974;**7**:45-78. Available from: http://link.springer.com/chapter/10.1007%2F978-1-4615-6944-2_2#page-1

[7] Margulis L. Symbiosis in Cell Evolution. Life and its Environment on the Early Earth. San Francisco: W. H. Freeman and Co; 1981. p. 415. Available from: http://onlinelibrary.wiley.com/doi/10.1002/jobm.19820220615/abstract

[8] Margulis L, Schwartz KV. Five Kingdoms. An Illustrated Guide to the Phyla of Life on Earth. 2nd ed. San Francisco: W. H. Freeman and Co; 1988. p. 376. Available from: https://www.jstor.org/stable/2413375?seq=1#page_scan_tab_contents

[9] Zernov DK. Essays of Phylogeny of Nonvascular Plantae. Kiev: Naukova dumka; 1972. p. 315 (in Russian)

[10] Odum EP, Odum HT. Fundamentals of Ecology. Philadelphia: W.B. Saunders; 1959. p. 400

[11] Odum E, Barrett GW. Fundamentals of Ecology. 5th ed. Belmont, Calif.: Thomson Brooks/Cole. 2005. p. 624. Available from: https://www.amazon.com/Fundamentals-Ecology-Eugene-Odum/dp/0534420664

[12] Kussakin OG, Drozdov AL. Phylema of the living beings. Part 1. Prolegomena to the Construction of Phylema. SPb.: Nauka; 1994. p. 272 (in Russian). Available from: http://bookoteka.ru/1_2_433.html

[13] Kussakin OG, Drozdov AL. Phylema of the living beings. Part 2. Prokaryotes, Eukaryotes: Microsporobiontes, Archaemonadobiontes, Euglenobiontes, Myxobiontes, Rhodobiontes, Alveolates, Heterokonts. SPb.: Nauka; 1998. p. 381 (in Russian). Available from: http://bookoteka.ru/1_2_433.html

[14] Jeffrey C. Thallophytes and kingdoms—A critique. Kew Bulletin. 1971;**25**:1-72. Available from: https://www.jstor.org/stable/4103226?seq=1#page_scan_tab_contents

[15] Jeffrey C. Kingdoms, codes and classification. Kew Bulletin. 1982;**37**:403-416. Available from: https://www.jstor.org/stable/4110040?seq=1#page_scan_tab_contents

[16] Leedale GF. How many are the Kingdoms of organisms? Taxon. 1974;**23**:261-270

[17] Edwards P. A classification of plants into higher taxa based on cytological and biochemical criteria. Taxon. 1976;**25**:529-542

[18] Ragan MA, Chapman A. Biochemical Phylogeny of the Protists. N.Y., San Francisco, L.: Academic Press; 1978. p. 317. Available from: https://books.google.ru/books?id=BqqnNKmU8I8C&pg=PA257&dq=Ragan+MA,+Chapman+A.+Biochemical+phylogeny+of+the+protists.+N.Y.,+San+Francisco,+L.&hl=ru&sa=X&ved=0ahUKEwja1JbS04HQAhUG8ywKHRZIClYQ6AEIVDAF#v=onepage&q=Ragan%20MA%2C%20Chapman%20A.%20Biochemical%20phylogeny%20of%20the%20protists.%20N.Y.%2C%20San%20Francisco%2C%20L.&f=false

[19] Starobogatov YI. The position of flagellated protists in the system of lower eukaryotes. Cytology (Цитология). 1995;**37**:1030-1037

[20] Möhn E. System und Phylogenie der Lebewesen. 1. Physikalisch-chemische und biologische Evolution, Procaryonta, Eucaryonta (bis Ctenophora). Stuttgart: Schweizerbart'sche Verlagsbuchhandlung; 1984. p. 884 S. Available from: http://www.schweizerbart.de/publications/detail/isbn/9783510651177/System_und_Phylogenie_der_Lebewesen

[21] Cavallier-Smith T. Kingdom protozoa and its 18 phyla. Microbiology Review. 1993;**57**: 953-994

[22] Cavallier-Smith T. Zooflagellate phylogeny and classification. Cytology (Цитология). 1995;**37**:1010-1029

[23] Cavallier-Smith T. A revised six-kingdom system of life. Biological Reviews of Cambridge Philosophical Society 1998;**73**:203-266. Available from: https://books.google.ru/books?id=-GyARbyTobYC&pg=PA158&dq=Cavallier-Smith+T.+A+revised+six-kingdom+system+of+life.+Biol.+Rev.+Comb.++Phylos.+Soc&hl=ru&sa=X&ved=0ahUKEwi1i_jQ1YHQAhWIdCwKHRn4BY8Q6wEIHzAA#v=onepage&q=Cavallier-Smith%20T.%20A%20revised%20six-kingdom%20system%20of%20life.%20Biol.%20Rev.%20Comb.%20%20Phylos.%20Soc&f=false

[24] Cavalier-Smith T. The phagotrophic origin of eukaryotes and phylogenetic classification of Protozoa. International Journal of Systematic and Evolutionary Microbiology. 2002;**52**:297-354. DOI: 10.1099/00207713-52-2-297

[25] Cavalier-Smith T. The neomuran origin of archaebacteria, the negibacterial root of the universal tree and bacterial megaclassification. International Journal of Systematic and Evolutionary Microbiology. 2002;**52**:7-76. Available from: http://www.microbiologyresearch.org/docserver/fulltext/ijsem/52/1/0520007a.pdf?expires=1477802129&id=id&accname=guest&checksum=93DC34728A09636A6C799F9529E111FC

[26] Vorontsov NN. Origin of life and diversity of its forms. Novosibirsk. 1965;55 (in Russian)

[27] Vorontsov NN. Systems of the organic world and the position of animals in them. 1. Russian Journal of Ecology. (Зоол. ж.). 1987;**66**:1668-1684 (in Russian)

[28] Vorontsov NN. Systems of the organic world and the position of animals in them. 2. Russian Journal of Ecology. (Зоол. ж.). 1987;**66**:1765-1774 (in Russian)

[29] Drozdov AL, Kussakin OG. State of the art and problems of megasystematics. In: Kryukov AP, editor. Problems of Evolution. Collected papers. **5**. Vladivostok: Dalnauka; 2003. pp. 18-30

[30] Drozdov AL. Multikingdom system of the living things. Russian Journal of Nematology. 2003;**11**(2):127-132

[31] Mashansky VF, Bobrova IF, Drozdov AL, Rizhamadze NA. The conservatism of membrane components of mitochondria. In: Troshin AS, editor. Structure and Function of Biological Membranes. Moskow.: Nauka; 1975. pp. 45-58 (in Russian)

[32] Mashansky VF, Drozdov AL. The principle of conservatism at the level of cellular ultrastructures and the problem of the appearance of life on Earth. In: Kull K, Tiivel T, editors. Lectures in Theoretical Biology. Tallinn: Valgus; 1988. pp. 113-120

[33] Mahler HR, Bastos RN, Feldman F, Urs FU, Lin Chi Chung, Perlman PhS, Sem H, Phan SH. Biogenetic autonomy of mitochondria and its limits. Some questions and new approaches to their answer. In: Tzagoloff A, editor. Membrane Biogenesis. Mitochondria, Chloroplasts, and Bacteria. New York, London: Plenum Press; 1975. pp. 15-61

[34] Cavalier-Smith T. Eukaryote kingdoms: Seven or nine? Bio-Systems. 1981;**14**:461-481. DOI: 10.1016/0303-2647(81)90050-2

[35] Cavalier-Smith T. A 6-kingdom classification and a unified phylogeny. In: Schwemmler W, Schenk HEH, editors. Endocytobiology. **2**. N.Y.: Walter de Gruyter & Co; 1983. pp. 1027-1034

[36] Cavalier-Smith T. Protist phylogeny and the high-level classification of Protozoa. European Journal of Protistology. 2003;**39**:338-348. DOI: 10.1078/0932-4739-00002

[37] Cavalier-Smith T. Only six kingdoms of life. Proceedings of the Royal Society. 2004;**271**:1251-1262. DOI: 10.1098/rspb.2004.2705

[38] Cavalier-Smith T. Deep phylogeny, ancestral groups and the four ages of life. Philosophical Transactions of the Royal Society B. 2010;**365**:111-132. DOI:10.1098/rstb.2009.0161

[39] Cavalier-Smith T. Early evolution of eukaryote feedingmodes, cell structural diversity, and classification of the protozoan phyla Loukozoa, Sulcozoa, and Choanozoa. European Journal of Agronomy. 2013;**49**:115-178. DOI: 10.1016/j.ejop.2012.06.001

[40] Shafranova LM. Plant as a life form. Journal of General Biology. (Ж. общ. биол.). 1990;**51**:72-88 (in Russian)

[41] Mirabdullaev IM. Problems of classification of a livings at the kingdom level. Journal of General Biology. (Ж. общ. биол.). 1989;**50**:725-736 (in Russian)

[42] Mirabdullaev IM. Problems of eukaryotes origin. Progress in Recent Biology (Успехи соврем. биол.). 1989;**107**:341-356 (in Russian)

[43] Christensen T. Algae: A Taxonomic Survey. Odense: AiO Print; 1980. Fasc. 1. p. 216

[44] Barr DJS. Evolution and kingdoms of organisms from the perspective of a mycologist. Mycologia. 1992;**84**;1-11

[45] Leontiev DV, Akulov AY. Revolution in megataxonomy: Prerequisites and results. Journal of General Biology (Ж. общ. биол.). 2002;**63**:168-186 (in Russian)

[46] Cavalier-Smith T. The kingdom chromista. In: Green JC, Leadbeater BSC, Diver WC, editors. The Chromophyte Algae: Problems and Perspectives. Oxford: Oxford University Press; 1989. pp. 379-405

[47] Fox GE, Stackebrandt E, Hespel RB, Gibson J, Maniloff J, Dyer TA, Wolfe RS, Balch WE, Tanner RS, Magrum LJ, Zablen LB, Gupta BRR, Bonen L, Lewis BJ, Stahl DA, Luehrsen KR, Chen KN, Woese CR. The phylogeny of prokaryotes. Science. 1980;**209**:457-463

[48] Woese CR, Fox GE. Phylogenetic structure of the prokaryotic domain: the primary kingdoms. Proceedings of the National Academy of Sciences of the United States. 1977;**74**: 5088-5090

[49] Woese CR. Bacterial evolution. Microbiology Review. 1987;**51**:221-271

[50] Woese CR, Kandler O, Wheelis ML. Toward a natural system of organisms: Proposal for the domains Archaea, Bacteria, and Eucarya. Proceedings of the National Academy of Sciences of the United States. 1990;**87**:4576-4579. DOI: 10.1073/pnas.87.12.4576

[51] Woese CR. A new biology for a new century. Microbiology and Molecular Biology Reviews. 2004;**68**:173-186. DOI:10.1128/MMBR.68.2.173-186.2004

[52] Woese CR, Goldenfeld N. How the microbial world saved evolution from the scylla of molecular biology and the charybdis of the modern synthesis. Microbiology and Molecular Biology Reviews. 2009;**73**(1):14-21. DOI: 10.1128/MMBR.00002-09

[53] Kandler O. Evolution of the systematic of bacteria. In: Schleifer KH, Stackebrand E. eds., Evolution of Prokaryotes. FEMS Symposium 29. L. etc: Academic Press; 1995. pp. 335-361

[54] Vossbrinck CR, Maddox JV, Friedman S, Debrunner-Vossbrinck BA, Woese CR. Ribosomal RNA sequence suggests microsporidia are extremely ancient eukaryotes. Nature. 1987;**326**:411-414

[55] Keeling PL, Fast NM. Microsporidia: Biology and evolution of highly reduced intracellular parasites. Annual Review of Microbiology. 2002;**56**:93-116. DOI: 10.1146/annurev.micro.56.012302.160854

[56] Gill EE, Fast NM. Assessing the microsporidia-fungi relationship: Combined phylogenetic analysis of eight genes. Gene. 2006;**375**:103-109

[57] Corradi N, Keeling PJ. Microsporidia: A journey through radical taxonomical revisions. Fungal Biology Review. 2009;**23**:1-8

[58] Corsaro D, Walochnik J, Venditti D, Steinmann J, Müller K-D, Michel R. Microsporidia-like parasites of amoebae belong to the early fungal lineage Rozellomycota. Parasitology Research. 2014;**113**. DOI: 10.1007/s00436-014-3838-4 Source: PubMed

[59] Capella-Gutiérrez S, Marcet-Houben M, Gabaldón T. Phylogenomics supports microsporidia as the earliest diverging clade of sequenced fungi. BMC Biology. 2012;**10**:47. Available from: http://www.biomedcentral.com/1741-7007/10/47. DOI: 10.1186/1741-7007-10-47

Chapter 2

Phylogenetics for Wildlife Conservation

José Luis Fernández-García

Additional information is available at the end of the chapter

http://dx.doi.org/10.5772/intechopen.69240

Abstract

Recent extinctions and the continuing threats to the survival of rare species will make conservation biology crucial in the twenty-first century. Conservation genetics for wildlife is an emerging challenge for humanity because it is accepted that a number of species and its populations are under oppression by a huge human expansion. Conservation genetics is the science that aims to minimize the risk of extinction. The International Union for Conservation of Nature and Natural Resources (IUCN) recognizes three hierarchical levels to conserve biodiversity: genetic diversity (populations), species (taxon ascertainment), and ecosystems (living organisms and their interactions). In view of the world's imminent biodiversity crisis, the risk of extinction at several biotic levels is nowadays unavoidable and requires urgent action. One prime conservation goal is focusing on preserving the genetic variation. The main reasons are: (1) to preserve a representation of past evolution and (2) to maintain raw material for future evolution, favoring the balance of ecosystems. Having these aims in mind, a new approach utilizes different metrics, such as phylogenetic diversity, split distance, and heightened evolutionary distinctiveness, which are being considered for immediate practical use to manage threat species and stocks submitted to new policies for conservation.

Keywords: distinctiveness metrics, extinction risk, genetics wildlife management, phylogenetic and conservation, species diversity

1. Introduction

> *"In the face of inevitable future losses to biodiversity, ranking species by conservation priority seems more than prudent. Setting conservation priorities within species (i.e., at the population level) may be critical as species ranges become fragmented and connectivity declines."* [1]

Ever since the revolutionary ideas put forward by Darwin, the evolutionary perspective of wildlife has played a fundamental role and has aimed to the efficient protection and preservation of biological diversity, which started off with an adequate, accurate or, at least, the best approached inventory of its current status. But the recent extinction or continuing threats to the disappearance of many species and populations has made conservation biology essential in the twenty-first century. The primary forces concerned with its long-term persistence of wildlife populations, may be ecological, political, economic, or other. Nowadays, these forces (or factors) use more objective genetics principles and related applications for conservation. In particular, the application of new molecular techniques, widely used in conservation research, has made genetics examination of endangered species feasible. Conservation genetics for wildlife is an emerging challenge for humanity because it is generally accepted that the extinction of present species, even some of its populations, were caused by the huge expansion of a sole species, the man (*Homo sapiens*). So, the number of studies based on genetic data aimed at understanding biological diversity patterns and processes has increased in recent years, partially, because biodiversity assessments made using species counts (e.g., total, endemic, threatened) may not be the most suitable metrics. In consequence, a more reliable approach has been proposed to improve the situation. On the one hand, using genetic data and phylogenetic analysis to adequately represent the processes that gave rise to the observed patterns of diversity and, on the other hand, allowing conservation efforts to apply not only to threatened species, but also to other particularly interesting populations. The metrics to be employed is yet under debate and an agreement needs to be reached.

As we said above, conservation genetics is the science that aims to minimize the risk of extinction from genetic factors [2]. Conservation genetics has flourished over the last 20 years and has shown that there are many ways genetic knowledge can help to conserve biodiversity, ranging from identifying the concerned populations to resolving taxonomic uncertainties, or understanding the biology of a focal taxon. The International Union for Conservation of Nature and Natural Resources (IUCN) is also focused on these ideas and recognizes three hierarchical levels to conserve biodiversity: genetic diversity (populations), species (taxon ascertainment), and ecosystems (living organisms and their interactions).

Although it is reasoned that endangered species have deserved a noteworthy attention on conservation research [3], less concerned species are also of research and sometimes conservation interest (e.g., European red deer [4, 5]). So, every species are important especially the distribution of their particular isolated populations when they are genetically distinct, although by not well known reasons. In this last case (including minor concern species), it reaches relevant importance to those inferior levels of taxonomic arrangement as subspecies, an historical nomination concept that is being replaced by evolutionary significant units (ESU), management units (MUs), and distinct population segments (DPS). In this way of thinking, the intraspecific diversity is officially recognized as one of three levels of biodiversity. This level of diversity, coupled with ecosystems and whole genetic diversity is worthy of protection [6] but often require more adequate information [7] about concerned species, ESUs, MU, or DPS [8].

In view of the world's imminent biodiversity crisis, referred to, by some people as the 'sixth mass extinction' but different from the five previous ones, "the next extinctions will be due to human impact", which are now unavoidable and need urgent actions to prevent it. Nowadays, optimistic scenarios predict significant changes in biodiversity around 2100, with most of the loss starting with isolated populations of whichever wild species.

http://dx.doi.org/10.5772/intechopen.69240

A large portion of the conservation genetics is dealing with the genetic conclusions about the causes and consequences of isolated small populations characterized by its low effective populations size (Ne), and simultaneously, the genetic drift effect because it causes a random change from generation to generation of gene pool. Whichever the case, they are both relevant issues associated to inbreeding under no random mating. The long-term effect of inbreeding leads to loss of genetic variability until reduced adaptability and ecosystem function, too [9].

Below the species level, it has been advocated the identification of populations that deserve long-term conservation or are derived from a recent rank fragmentation [10–12]. Although populations' relationships are being represented by bifurcating trees, it is known that bifurcating trees often fail to show everything and/or complex relationships, a major shortcoming if populations do need to be prioritized for conservation [1]. In this way of thinking, several studies have shown how measuring and maximizing phylogenetic diversity can be performed using phylogenetic networks and evolutionary isolation indices adapted for populations within species ([1, references therein). The new approach utilizes different metrics, like phylogenetic diversity (PD), split distance (SD) [13], or Shapley metric (SH) [14], and heightened evolutionary distinctiveness (HED) (refined by [15]) to assess not only from the species level, but also to population differentiations within each other. These metric might be of immediate practical use to manage discrete populations within species with several degrees of threat and stocks submitted to new policies for conservation triage [16].

2. The phylogenetic context

The concepts of taxonomy are familiar for every biologist because they have spent a long time studying species names and retrospectively their order into genus, family, ..., kingdoms. Such a classification recalls a scenario like ancestor-descendent relationships among taxa (phylogeny), which result in a scheme describing an evolutionary relationship that could not be subject to critical analysis. Recently, modern phylogenetic science captures, as empirically as possible, the relatedness among similar taxa using the most orderly manner for mapping the path of evolution that leads to and represents the true ancestry relating the upstream organisms. The resultant classification must be reasonably and objectively assumed by worldwide biologists, undoubtedly. In this way, groups of species or its populations are essentially related by a set of both, morphological and molecular characteristics but, more importantly yet, these should be matched by properties such as its ecological abilities.

Firstly, phylogenetic studies have been proven to be of utility, of course, but in a research-oriented framework. In this way, a simple data research can provide guidelines to find gaps and strengthen interpretations to ensure management affirmations. So, multi-locus phylogenies can be used to infer the species tree whose nodes represent the actual separation between species, thus providing essential information about their evolutionary history or helping analyzes of species delimitation, gene flow, and genetic differentiation within species [17]. As an example, now adequate markers are available by extracting intron information from genomes of human, chimpanzee, macaque, cow, and dog (three mammalian orders) searching for the

ENSEMBL database. This analysis led to a final list of 224 intron markers randomly distributed along the genome for six mammals species, which can be useful to gather genetic markers with unambiguous phylogenetic signals (see [17] for details and design) (**Figure 1**).

Secondly, the use of phylogenetic diversity is of current interest in view of its objective metrics for conservation in evolution history (the past), genetic status of species (the present), and

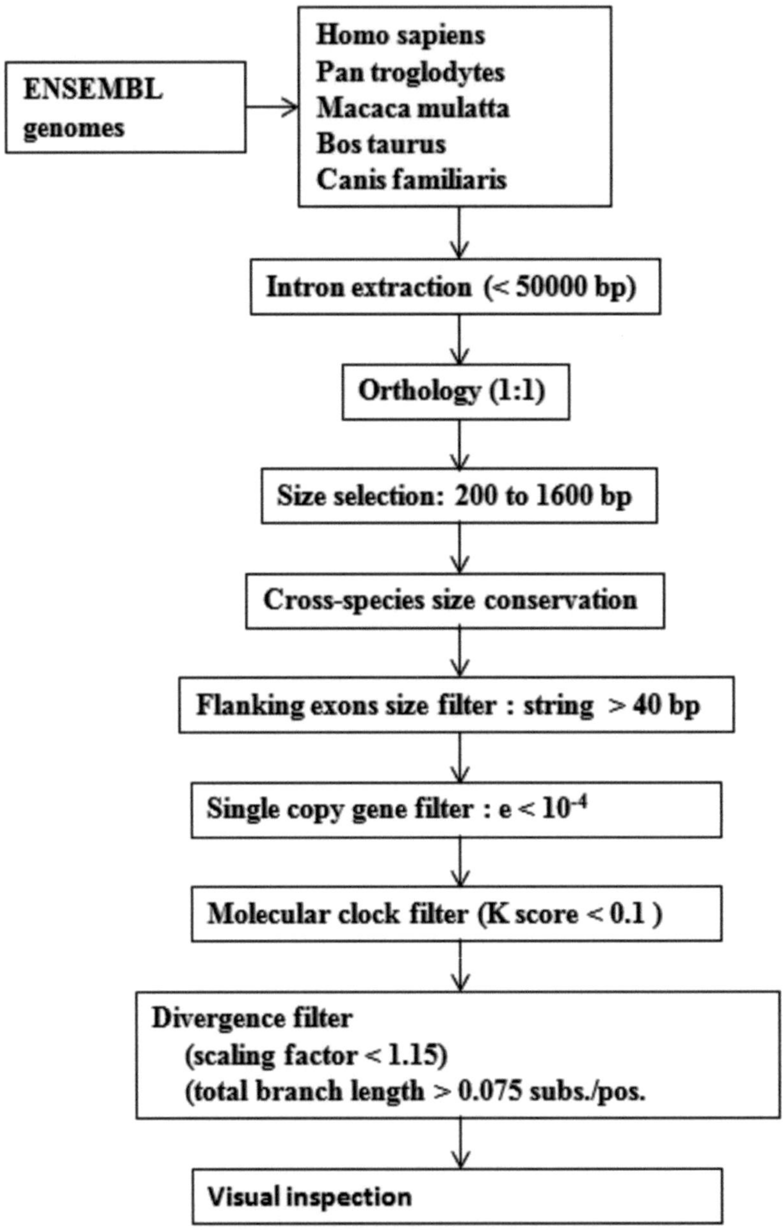

Figure 1. Steps for intron extractions and filtering processes. Adapted from [17].

http://dx.doi.org/10.5772/intechopen.69240

management for conservation in geographically split species (the future).The first two may be of general interest on research, but within a practical approach the last issue is of plentiful applicability to wildlife population management. The phylogenetic ramifications reflect more than simple systematic classifications. The molecular information and its association with other kinds of data can be an objective measure to identify species or population groups with different or similar vital aptitude such as habitat use among taxa or similar facts. A straightforward example has been pointed out in the case of strong associations between habitats and morphology in shorebirds, ducks, and other water bird species. However, supposedly described subspecies differentiation (e.g., the specimens of the whole geographic Iberian range was pooled as a single genetic population instead of delimiting them as lineage clusters) based on morphological information has been seen to fail, probably due to the mixing of genetic lineages. After a molecular survey of the Iberian desman (*Galemys pyrenaicus*), the data set suggested two main phylogenetic clusters delimited by mitochondrial DNA (**Figure 2**) in this emblematic species. Because of a strong geographic splitting in type localities of this species and the absence of clear morphological discrimination with nowadays data, its populations may easily be regrouped in two big clades that would correspond to two nominal subspecies *Galemys pyrenaicus rufulus* (clade A) and *Galemys pyrenaicus pyrenaicus* (clade B) [18]. Consequently, it has recently been suggested to treat these outstanding lineages as separated groups in the wildlife management contexts.

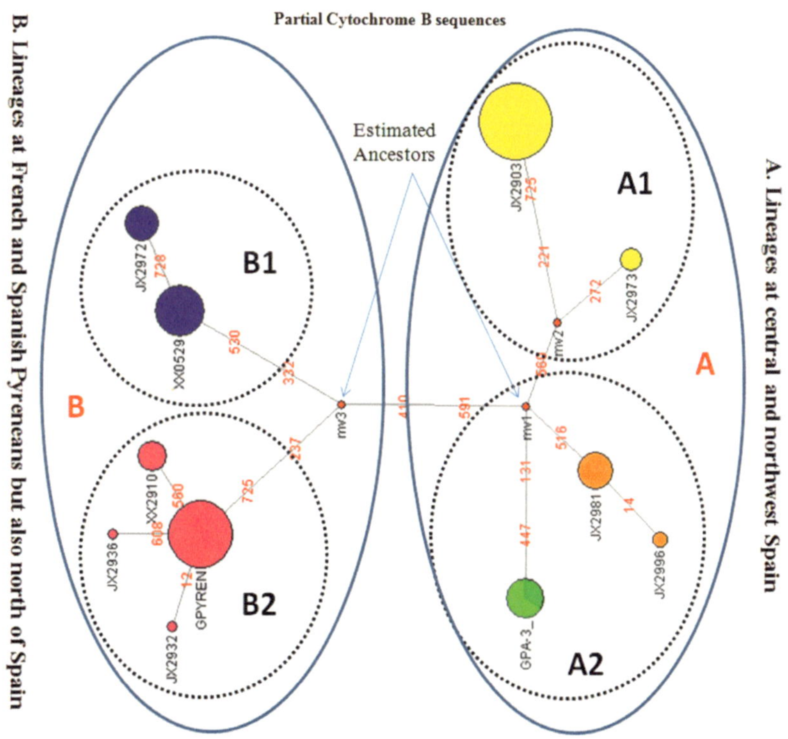

Figure 2. Main lineages in *Galemys pyrenaicus*. Adapted from [18].

Thirdly, however, is the issue of hybridization: a cause for debate. Hybridizations have occurred for long and they are well known by managers and scientists around the world. The main question about hybridization is which, the species or its hybrid, should be prioritized and valued. The concept of hybridization understood to mean mating between different species has been extended to mating between two genetically distinct populations that produce offspring (F1 to several backcross; **Figure 3**), regardless of its fertility.

Two competing effects of such introgression are assumed but with different final results on species diversity: (1) **a negative view** is a feeling of concern when human activity is the main cause of the introgression [19] and (2) **a positive view** is when nature is the main responsible of admixture among populations but with a long-term component [20] because, at present, man intervention is in everything, so, consequently, the first view is the one that is considered of most concern.

One well-studied example about the negative effect of human impact on hybridization in wildlife in nonthreatened species is the European red deer. During the last century (past and currently also), there has been an extensive arbitrary trading of European red deer aimed at breeding improved trophies for hunting on extinct or nearly extinct autochthonous populations [21]. The direct consequence of the restocking and the action of introducing genetically-distinct populations has had various types of negative effects. On the one hand, hybridization with introduced animals has impaired the phylogenetic boundaries between former and natural populations, contributing to blurring true genetic history and confounding future researches. Worldwide allochthonous and indigenous red deer have been admixed (and are) through several Europe countries. It is believed that the scarce documentation about this fact is opposite to the true dimension of human impact, which should have been huge instead. Because of a generalized worldwide impact of anthropic action, a mixture of phylogenetic scenarios would probably be expected (**Figure 4**). Accordingly, though genetic variation is supposedly structured hierarchically, some exceptions occurred under hybridization associated to human activity. To overcome this drawback, an effective sampling strategy according to the specific problem should be design based on knowledge. In the European red deer example, due to the arbitrariness of admixture, these scenarios caused different effects. One of them may be the presence of mixture allochthonous lineages as in Val di Susa (Italy) being genetically similar to Bulgarian red deer. Although the origin of Val di Susa red deer was

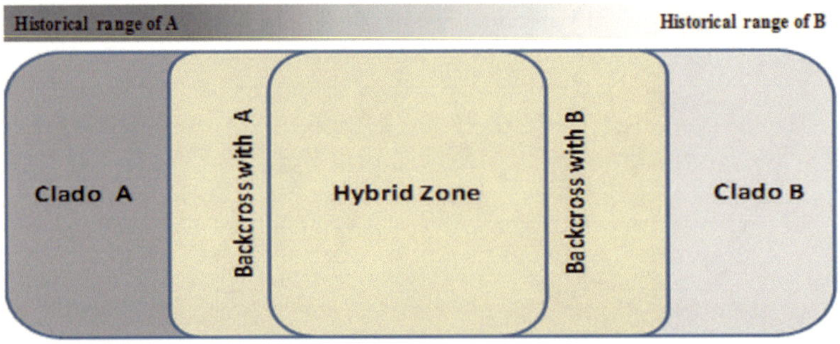

Figure 3. The most probable distribution of hybrid and their backcross in a natural framework of admixture.

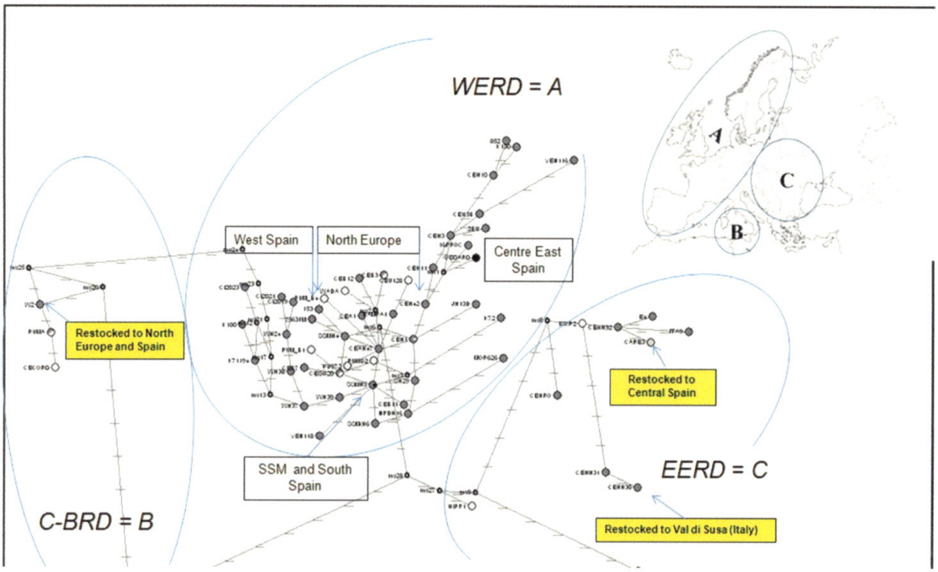

Figure 4. Phylogeography scenario of European red deer lineages. A = "Western European red deer" lineages, B = C-BRD "Corsican and Barbary red deer" lineages, and C = ERRD "Eastern European red deer" lineages. Map showing natural geography distribution of lineages. Network showed some restocked lineages into different areas of Spain and Europe (yellow quadrate).

Slovenia and Bulgaria; only Bulgarian blood survived, probably attributed to genetic drift. But in this case, the population could be easily qualified as allochthonous. On the other hand, outbreeding depression of the hybrid offspring due to lower reproductive success or survival of either parent has also been found. In our example, translocation of Wapitis and Asian red deer (today regarded as different species from European red deer) was unsuccessful by far, as a way to result in antler-size improvement. This failure was partially due to the **lack of adaptation** to local environmental factors or high susceptibility to local diseases. This example suggested outbreeding depression in hybrid populations [21]. Two mechanisms have been proposed for the outbreeding depression. An **intrinsic mechanism** upholds a reduced fitness of hybrids due to interactions between genes originating in different evolutionary taxa. Conversely, **extrinsic mechanisms** advocated for loss of adaptation to local environment with unsuccessful reproduction. Also, the interaction genotype-environment may be assessed.

Moreover, hybridized populations or species may consist on a hybrids swarm in which all individuals are to various degrees of admixture. In this respect, an important role in transferring or restocking species or populations to the wild is being played by enclosures (in zoos or collections), which serve as reservoirs of different populations and subspecies. Sometimes, these reservoirs have acted as the origin of feral populations of many different exotic species and subspecies contaminating autochthonous stocks. This was the case of the Woburn red deer from Bedfordshire [21] or the Mesopotamian fallow deer at the Opel Zoo [22]. In the latter case, phylogenetic studies can be used to assay the presence of hybridization in the Persian fallow deer from the Israeli Reintroduction Program started in 1996 and thus dispel all doubts.

The positive side of hybridization is more related to speciation. Hybridization occurs more frequently than previously recognized and is an important source of speciation. Hybridization leading to a new taxon, distinct from both parent species, is called (when homoploid) hybrid speciation or recombinational speciation [23]. Almost 50% of plant species originated from the hybridization of different species. For example, 10% of bird species are believed to hybridize with another species naturally. This sort of speciation promoted adaptive divergence and increased reproductive isolation. But introgressed genetic variation can also enhance the ability to coexist and promote invasiveness [24] enlarging the range of a hybrid populations. Moreover, a positive feedback between hybridization and speciation may exist [25]. So, hybridization may increase (1) the rate of speciation, (2) diversity of closely related species, and (3) adaptive radiation by incorporation into populations of selectively favored alleles or combinations of them; providing the basis for adaptive evolution and having important implications for the origin of new species.

The frequency of hybridization as a source of adaptive variation for speciation may be summarized as follows: firstly, hybridization among species occur about 10–30% of multicellular species regularly on a per-species basis but less frequently on a per-individual basis, the latter more frequently driven by humans (as the case of *Dama dama mesopotamica* described in [22]). Secondly, mutations are rare, around 10^{-8} to 10^{-9} per generation per base pair, that is, a considerable time for novel adaptations to appear but depending also on the population size. So, hybridization among species can act as a source of adaptive genetic variation rather than mutation [26–30]. For example, 'New additive genetic variance introduced by hybridization in Darwin's finches, which has been estimated to be two to three orders of magnitude greater than that introduced by mutation' [26], despite initial hybridization itself, which is unlikely to be adaptive because there is often evidence of selected against. Last but not least, adaptation is thought to be the most important process driving divergence during speciation [31–33] and divergence in ecology occurs almost exclusively under selection. Moreover, closely related species tend to hybridize more often. Species in rapidly diversifying adaptive radiations could especially be prone to hybridization [25, 34, 35].

3. Conservation genetics

Conservation genetics was born in the last third of the twentieth century integrating empirical and theoretical studies based on population genetic data, which were incorporated to the Conservation Biology doctrine giving rise to the discipline "Conservation Genetics" with a spectacular growth. The conceptual framework included all "genetics" issues that are phylogenetic, quantitative, evolutionary, ecological, and population genetics themes.

Nowadays, conservation genetics is being applied for practical conservation and wildlife management as a major paradigm. At first, the conservation of species was evaluated by indirect and phenotypic data but powerful advances on DNA technology resulted in a huge amount of genetic data more easily achieved, and also helped by an emerging sophisticated statistical procedures. Now, it is possible to gather the objective information coded long ago into genomes of every organism. Thereafter, the conservation genetic discipline raised its interest

http://dx.doi.org/10.5772/intechopen.69240

when people became aware of the growing rate of human population and its unavoidable effect on planet biodiversity. The IUCN (World Conservation Union, formerly International Union for Conservation of Nature diversity either ecosystems or species) recognized three main levels worthy of protection and conservation: genetic diversity within species, species in themselves, and either local or global ecosystems. However, the first goal in the mind of conservation geneticist is the assessments of genetic variability in threatened and unthreatened organisms as a metric to trace the well-being of the planet.

3.1. Relevant items in conservation genetics: wildlife scenario from top to bottom

3.1.1. Kinship and genetic variation for within population conservation (population genetics)

The loss of genetic variation due to inbreeding (as a result of mating among genetically related individuals) was (and is yet) the main issue regarding captive and natural populations of small size. Whichever the case, despite great scientific attention received by the deleterious effects arising from inbreeding depression; no less important are parentage, kinship, sex identification, and demographic history of population. Since a general scientific acknowledgement regarding inbreeding depression related to small captive populations and natural isolated populations as well, a preference position has been granted to those studies focused on inbreeding depression. The assessing of inbreeding depression has been the former issue in the design of conservation programs, formerly applied to domestic animals and plants, but today it has been extended to wildlife, both in captive breeding programs and in the management of natural isolated populations. An interesting case is the Pyrenean desman (*G. pyrenaicus*), which is annotated as vulnerable by the IUCN red list. However, the southernmost population in the Iberian peninsula (at the mountain place of the central system: green dashes in **Figure 2**) is listed as "endangered" with high extinction risk by the main Spanish government authority (MAGRAMA, that is, Ministry of Agriculture, Food and Environment) due to its almost null genetic variation (mtDNA studies suggested they carried a clonal lineage in several populations) and high level of anthropic threat but without possibility of implementing captive breeding programs [18].

Regarding population variations in wildlife, it is important to assess local kinship as offspring parentage, mating systems, sex determination, or lineages identification. The main field of study is the application of empirical data to be compared with theoretical assumptions as in the case of diploid lethal equivalents estimation to juvenile survival [36]. New DNA technologies are addressing molecular procedures to gather high informative loci as microsatellites and single nucleotide polymorphisms (SNPs) to finely estimate relatedness coefficient at several degrees of relatives, not only to parents-offspring pairs. An underestimate of the total impact of inbreeding has been declared and Ne/N bias between nonbreed and unmanaged wild population has been claimed after assuming statistical distribution of family size (Poisson distribution). The relative importance of the analysis of local kinships has several issues as follows: (i) isolated populations differ by drift and inbreeding but the first is more related to random sampling than specifically mating of relatives; (ii) balance among family sizes can be calculated by molecular procedures using as many genetic markers as possible in local or isolated populations; (iii) local populations exhibited correlations between diversity and family sizes but unbalances in this last one may influence minimum viable populations size(MVPs) (number of individuals needed for long-term persistence of populations with high probability), which assist scientific and wildlife managers in population viability analysis (PVA). However, some discrepancies arose between theoretical and empirical studies comparison about the deleterious effect of inbreeding, suggesting a case-by-case analysis in wild species due to strong species specific conditionings: lifestyle, demographic history, genetics, and more. Other significant assessment related to conservation is heterozygosity. It may be useful to understand a species life history. This type of analysis allows us to give a retrospective look at the past to make current comparisons and to perform realistic predictions about the future.

3.1.2. Conservation genetic of geographic variation

Ecological and evolutionary sources of genetic variation, at the intra-specific level or higher, are also worth of being considered for conservation purposes. However, the two main areas of work in this broad field of study have its top representatives in phylogeography and genetics of populations. These two approaches are being used currently, one based on allelic frequencies (unordered polymorphism for population genetics but recently also phylogeography using e.g., network-net methods) and the other one based on mitochondrial DNA sequences (ordered polymorphism for phylogeography also using networks as in **Figure 4**). Both approaches are utilized because they can easily represent the pattern of spatial distribution of genetic variation for species and allocate the most genetically isolated populations and connectedness degree if any. Moreover, there is a current tendency to rejoin historical genealogical information plus contemporary forces modeling populations because it is believed to provide a larger resolution to illuminate the causes and consequences of such spatial pattern in nature. Moreover, practical biodiversity conservation is interested in conserving as many species or relevant populations within them allocated inside emblematic or unique places following the "species' genetic richness" concept.

At least, three competing concepts that connect researchers on conservation genetics and conservation managers, also needing to be delimited in the conservation biology context, are those that follow: evolutionary significant units (ESUs), managements units (MUs), and phylogenetic diversity (PD) of taxa as a way to estimate distinct population segments (DPS) [1]. Today, these three concepts are fully applicable for wildlife analysis and to take relevant decisions. The idea of MUs should be seen regardless of how recent the prior genetic history connections was, providing that exchange of individuals is so small as to be demographically independent units. By contrast, ESUs must imply a long historical separation of its populations. However, approaches based on demography and connectedness between populations can treat species or populations unequally. Consequently, a new appraisal introduces evaluations of phylogenetic trees connecting species (or populations within species) under a study approach called "Phylogenetic Diversity of taxa" (PDs). This approach has into account the edge length distances of the tree. Edge lengths depict the optimal number of features uniquely shared by all descending taxa below this edge and using a root. The set of taxa (populations) that maximizes the PD (normally less than the total populations considered) could be utilized in two types of projects. It has been employed to identify taxa and/or populations prone for conservation purposes. On the other hand, it is also a way to identify important taxa or geographically isolated for sequencing projects.

3.1.3. *Biodiversity of species*

In this section, the basic idea is that unique evolutionary lineages may contribute largely to overall genetics diversity. Their extinction would constitute a far great loss of diversity than would the extinction of species that have extant close relative. Although under discussion, phylogenetic distinctiveness is dealing with resolution of taxonomic issues due to its recognized role as measurement of taxon worthy of investing conservation resources. It is generally admitted that the importance of research to delineate the influence of introgression and hybridization on species diversity. It is a topic that is reaching great relevance at the inter-specific level but also at the inter-subspecific level as a way of **silent extinction** due to human domestication of current wild species and random translocation of their products, overriding yet hidden evolutionary pathways unexpectedly by introgressive extinction (as for red deer subspecies, **Figure 4**).

In this state of things, the systematic evaluation focusing on elevating differentiated populations such as true species assessed by informative genetic loci of split populations. This is an important issue for wildlife conservation and for making management decisions. Several subspecies gathered the rank of species (e.g., historical nominal subspecies as Wapiti but today elevated to the species level: *Cervus canadensis* instead of *Cervus elaphus canadensis*) or at least will be considered from this point worth of deepest studies as Mesopotamian fallow deer (*Dama dama mesopotamica*) or Barbary red deer (*Cervus elaphus barbarus*), which are currently included in their respective conservation programs or even herdbooks. Hopefully, conservation programs and the creation of herdbooks to manage the most endangered species should be treated as a nonnegligible new Genetic discipline: "Domestic" wildlife issue. Nevertheless, it should not be obviate that the rate of speciation, diversity of closely related species and adaptive radiation by incorporation into populations of selectively favorable alleles or combinations of them may be increased by hybridization, providing thus, the basis for adaptive evolution and having important implications for the origin of species, as mentioned previously.

3.1.4. *Wildlife forensic: the case of Pyrenean desman in ecological studies*

Forensic identification by advanced DNA technology is also important for wildlife studies. But forensic analysis has several distinct fields of application. Firstly, free-ranging wildlife species, especially those endangered, where noninvasive methods are recommended to detect elusive or sensitive to human management species as sampling strategies (e.g., Pyrenean desman (*G. pyrenaicus*)). On the other hand, wildlife products from specimens under strict police management due to them are imperiled (e.g., rhinoceros horns).

Finally, the biology and ecology of species with elusive or with hidden activity, which are still poorly known. As an example, the nature of trophic interactions is a fundamental issue in ecology and has aroused the attention of biologists for decades. This knowledge is particularly important in endangered species such as the Pyrenean desman. Using DNA from feces of the Pyrenean desman, it is possible to identify 19 prey species by next generation sequencing methods like the DNA minibarcode (133 bp) of the COI gene barcoding. This tool is able to simultaneously perform screening of species at large-scale because sometimes feces could be difficult to identify directly. Despite potential pitfalls in this methodology, it is based on one or a few genes at present state, each new genome incorporated into the data bank increases the validity of it. Consequently, more and more literature is arising in recent times.

4. Biodiversity analysis by integrating phylogeny and conservation

Quantification of biodiversity using phylogenetic analyzes has been proposed to provide a more objective framework to make conservation decisions. Three collaborative efforts among ecologists, evolutionary biologists, paleontologists, systematists, and conservation biologists from the USA, Canada, Australia, and England are driving these aims thorough the 'Tree of Life' project attempting to integrate phylogenetic and conservation biology. They are based on two complementary facts: (1) surprising amounts of phylogenetic diversity might remain even under high rates of extinction (random) and (2) it is feasible to detect current extinction events through missing phylogenetic diversity as it is mentioned in [37].

Three issues are being examined in the integrative framework as follow:

4.1. Selectivity or random extinctions questions: species or upper taxonomic level

The start viewpoint of New and May's was that simulated extinction occurred at random with respect to phylogeny [37]. However, phylogeny and conservation working groups ('phylogeny and conservation' working group sponsored by the National Center for Ecological Analysis and Synthesis (NCEAS) in Santa Barbara, CA, USA) reasoned that in this context randomness is not realistic due to extinctions and invasions tend to be strongly clumped for the most diverse taxonomic groups, for example, mammals or birds. After testing several statistics by simulation, the Moran's *I* index showed the high performance for detecting selectivity accurately, independent of tree size (i.e., number of species), tree shape (i.e., nodes with equal size groups in the tree), or prevalence of the desired trait (e.g., proportion of endangered or invasive species). As a result, it has been recognized that taxonomic selectivity is the main way to extinction and could be quantified, but hopefully selectivity varies across a wide variety of taxonomic groups, across geographical regions, between 'higher' and 'lower' taxonomic units, and extinction is related to selectivity for invasion within taxonomic groups.

4.2. Levels below species

A long-standing problem is how to designate conservation units below the species level: Subspecies, ESUs, MUs, and more. With the advent of molecular technologies, those historical concepts as "subspecies" fell in disuse. However, an overload of genetic information can lead to the designation of many small and isolated subunits hampering the standard delimitation of, for example, the ESU and MUs concepts. A survey of the recent literature revealed that most studies follow the guidelines of Moritz, which advocate a purely genetic definition of ESUs. Nevertheless, a large fraction of conservation decisions require both genetic and ecological evidence.

The guidelines of Moritz admitted that ESUs should show significant divergence and reciprocal monophyly for mtDNA and significant divergence of allele frequencies at nuclear loci. This is straightforward because it requires to examine historical and recent restrictions to gene flow, that is, evidence for long-term divergence that continued in the mtDNA and nuclear loci (free from selection) where mutations accumulate relatively more slowly or very rapidly, respectively. Therefore, this molecular discrepancy is useful to evaluate restrictions to gene flow at different times or even detecting genetic distinctiveness but no adaptive potential. However, Moritz's definition no-longer mentions the ecological distinctness because ecological divergence may or may not be necessarily associated to genetic divergence. Crandall et al. [8] proposed the "cross-hair analysis" to have into account the four important scenarios to decide whether ESUs or not is present (**Figure 5**).

Consequently, there is a worldwide agreement that decisions should be based on both genetic and ecological evidence but in the context of ecological and genetic exchangeability. Ecology together with an examination of recent and historical processes provide a more fine-grained, and therefore, more flexible categorization than the current system to be employed to diverse set "case studies" as red wolf (*Canis rufus*), dusky seaside sparrow (*Ammodramus maritimus nigrescens*), Florida panther (*Puma concolor coryi*), and Gila topminnow (*Poeciliopsis occidentalis occidentalis*) or Pyrenean desman (*G. pyrenaicus*).

4.3. Areas with distinct population segments (DPS): hotspots places

There are many criteria to determine the relative conservation value of different areas (e.g., species, threatened species or large numbers of species across different groups), but now below species level as areas containing DPS received attention since the late 1980s mainly for economic-important taxa. The problem is how we can quantify DPS value. Population-based management is being a necessary task for scientists and managers due to climate change and habitat degradation associated to growing human demands ensuring continued species-range fragmentation, which will be expected during this century. In order to address this work, phylogenetic diversity (PD) is being used as a measure of at least three stuffs to choose important areas to protect with accountability incorporating phylogenetic information.

Firstly, the exploration of the relations between PD and the spatial distribution of biodiversity would permit to get insight into the population structure complementary to the current statistical assessment of differentiation employed by MUs and DPS. Moreover, under this perspective, it is feasible, when constrained, to choose only a limited number of areas for conservation, to develop appropriate protocols to assess the complementarity predictions to preserve future biodiversity. Secondly, PD is being extended to simulations aimed to find taxonomically nonrandom extinction risk. Current threat scenarios are tested by comparing the spatial distribution of PD both before and after projected extinction. Finally, the predictions that suggest rapid environmental change leads to explore whether phylogenetic patterns of threat could predict the amount of ecological disturbance in a region.

+reject H_0 of exchangeability, evidence exists for divergence.
-accept H_0 of exchangeability, failure to detect divergence.

		Time Frame
+/-	+/-	Recent
+/-	+/-	Ancient
Genetic divergence	Ecological divergence	
H_0Exchangeability		

Figure 5. Cross-hair analysis for management recommendations (adapted from [8]).

5. Prioritizing populations for conservation using phylogenetic distances from networks: split diversity (SD)

According to the "species richness" concept [38], practical biodiversity conservation has the aim to preserve as many species as possible. However, as previously said, such an approach has the hurdle of treating all species equally [39]. However, neither all species nor genetic lineages are equally important, with more isolated lineages providing more important contribution to total variation, that is, the base for identifying populations worthy of protection in law. Genetic variation is depicted perfectly onto a rooted phylogenetic tree, where the edge length represents the number of features uniquely shared by all descending taxa, say populations. Importantly, ESUs concept assumes that the relationships among populations can be represented by a bifurcating tree. However, these sort of phylogenetic trees often fail to capture complete genetic information among populations. Moreover, more complex interrelationships are expected for DPSs and MUs. So, it would seem a shortcoming could occur if populations do need to be prioritized for conservation on the basis of tree-based prioritization schemes. However, the prioritization approaches for trees can also be adapted for populations by using algorithms developed for network under the denomination "Neighbor-Net" procedures [1], where PD could be optimized via computing a circular split system. Optimal PD could be obtained by morphological and molecular data. Using PD, Faith [40] proposed a taxa selection once having a phylogenetic tree of n taxa by identifying the set of k taxa that maximizes the PD, where $k < n$. The optimal set is tested yet to determine taxa that are of interest for sequencing projects in wildlife [41]. Although mathematical formulations exceeded our aims, following [13] we summarize the example in the paper of these authors to show how it works.

In **Figure 6**, we show a network graph ordered in a circular format A to E taxon. Each split could be weighted according to edge distances from each bisecting taxon (arrows in **Figure 6**) to the rest of taxa. As an example, the procedure to get an optimal PD distance (PD is equivalent to SD in Ref. [13]) form circular taxon order of A–E will be constructed for an optimal three-set of split taxon as follows:

(i) Formulae to be used (n°4 in [13]).

(ii) Compute the pairwise distance matrix d_{uv} (distance count).

http://dx.doi.org/10.5772/intechopen.69240

	A	B	C	D	E
A	0	11	19	20	17
B	11	0	12	21	22
C	19	12	0	17	18
D	20	21	17	0	11
E	17	22	18	11	0

(iii) Index matrix to trace back the optimum. The 3-Path taxon maximizing DP (in blue an example: the ABC maximum 3-path DP; see **Figure 6**).

		A	B	C	D	E
	A			B	C	C
	B				C	D
α^3_{uv} =	C					D
	D					
	E					

(iv) Compute the longest ordered two-path using $L^2 = d_{uv}$ (as in second line at formulae).

		A	B	C	D	E
	A		11	19	20	17
	B			12	21	22
L^2 =	C				17	18
	D					11
	E					

(v) Derived L^3 from L^2 (as in second line at formulae) but only three taxa.

Example A to C = (3+2+4+2) + (2+6+4) = 23 (B features two times¡)

Example B to E = (2+4+6+4+5) + (5+2+4) = 32

		A	B	C	D	E
	A			23	36	37
	B				29	32
L^3 =	C					28
	D					
	E					

(vi) Calculate $L^3 + L^2$ for the longest ordered three-path.

		A	B	C	D	E
	A			42	56	54
	B				50	54
$L^3 + L^2 =$	C					46
	D					
	E					

(vii) Determine maximal scores SD max (three-circular tour) as $(L^3 + L^2)_{max}$ =56/2.

(viii) Determine the longest ordered three-path from A to D using α^3_{uv}. As a result, the set ACD is an element SD_3 with the highest scores for $PD_3 = 28$.

Several phylogenetic diversity measures have been adapted for nontree-like population genetic data. However, these methods could be conditioned to change when natural or artificial (human mediated) extinction alters the network structure. Given both the stochastic and/or selective nature of extinction, different metrics, like split diversity (SD; similar to PD) from [13] or Shapley metric (SH [14]), and heightened evolutionary distinctiveness (HED [15]) offer general ranking systems useful to wildlife managers rather than those based only on the present structure of a phylogenetic network trees. However, SH and HED rankings have been stated as able to allow lengthening or shortening the list of taxa to conserve in the event that resources become more or less available, which may give potential relevant frameworks or schemes for preserving future biodiversity [1].

split		Mutation weight or "features"
A	BCDE	3
B	ACDE	2
C	ABDE	4
D	ABCE	5
E	ABCD	4
AB	CDE	6
BC	ADE	4
CD	ABE	2
DE	ABC	4

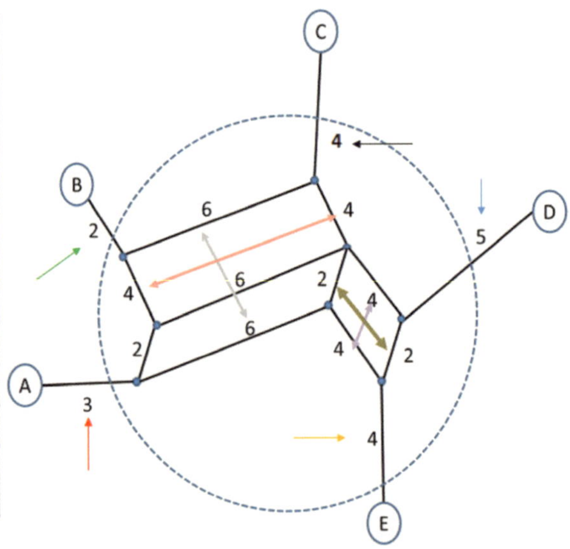

Figure 6. Split graph and its split systems (adapted from [13]).

Nowadays, the most recent, more inexpensive, and robust advances in molecular techniques make of the genetic sampling of populations a standard component of conservation planning. Moreover, there are views that value phylogenetic network approach because it offers insight into a species' population structure complementary to the current statistical assessments of differentiation employed by MUs and DPSs [11, 12]. Genotyping at multiple informative loci and networks will provide population genetic studies aimed at giving advice to conservation agencies, to do more informative and accurate estimates of population differentiation and of conservation-relevant processes, mainly those important onto genetic isolation and their effects on diversity [42].

6. Conclusion

Conservation genetics for wildlife is a recent challenge for humanity because biodiversity at several biotic levels need to be preserved to maintain desirable genetic variation for future generations. As a result, understanding biological diversity patterns and processes has increased the interest for phylogenetic analysis, remaining relevant all species. Nowadays, the imminent biodiversity crisis predicts significant new scenarios of biodiversity at the beginning of the twenty-second century for whichever wild species, which motivates to the geneticists in deal with preserve "all the gene pool". However, two faced situations are clearly involved in the context of conservation decisions. On the one hand, the identification of small populations harbors any significant genetic relevance worthy of conservation. On the other hand, identification of natural hybridized populations or species, although do not lack detractors when artificially promoted, due to it is believed to be an important process causing divergence in speciation and enhances the ability for survive. So, practical biodiversity conservation has the aim to preserve as many species (populations) as possible, but the relative importance of species or its genetic lineages should be carefully studied for to be prioritized. Phylogenetic diversity measures have been adapted to offer potential relevant frameworks or schemes for preserving future biodiversity based on accurate estimates of population differentiation and conservation processes.

Author details

José Luis Fernández-García

Address all correspondence to: pepelufe@unex.es

Genetic and Animal Breeding, Animal Production Department. Faculty of Veterinary. Universidad de Extremadura, Cáceres, Spain

References

[1] Volkmann L, Martyn I, Moulton V, Spillner A, Mooers AO. Prioritizing populations for conservation using phylogenetic networks. PLoS One. 2014;**9**(2):e88945. DOI: 10.1371/journal.pone.0088945

[2] Pemberton J. Introduction to conservation genetics. In: Frankham R, Ballou JD, Briscoe DA. Genetical Research. Cambridge University Press. 2004;**83**(3):221-222. DOI: 10.1017/S0016672304216913

[3] Hedrick PW. Conservation genetics: Where are we now?. Trends in Ecology and Evolution. 2001;**16**:629-636. DOI: 10.1016/S0169-5347(01)02282-0

[4] Fernández-García JL, Carranza J, Martínez JG, Randi E. Mitochondrial D-loop phylogeny signals two native Iberian red deer (*Cervus elaphus*) Lineages genetically different to Western and Eastern European red deer and infers human-mediated translocations. Biodiversity and Conservation. 2014;**23**(3): 537-554. DOI: 10.1007/s10531-013-0585-2

[5] Zachos FE, Frantz AC, Kuehn R, Bertouille S, Colyn M, et al. Genetic structure and effective population sizes in European red deer (*Cervus elaphus*) at a Continental scale: Insights from microsatellite DNA. Journal of Heredity. 2016;**107**(4):318-326. DOI: 10.1093/jhered/esw011

[6] Zachos FE. Gene trees and species trees—Mutual influences and interdependences of population genetics and systematics. Journal of Zoological Systematics and Evolutionary Research. 2009;**47**:209-218. DOI: 10.1111/j.1439-0469.2009.00541.x

[7] Soulé ME. What is conservation biology? BioScience. 1985;**35**:727-734. DOI: 10.2307/1310054

[8] Crandall KA, Bininda-Emonds OR, Mace GM, Wayne RK. Considering evolutionary processes in conservation biology. Trends in Ecology and Evolution. 2000;**15**(7):290-295. DOI: 10.1016/S0169-5347(00)01876-0

[9] Redding DW, Mooers AØ. Can systematists help decide the relative worth of bits of biodiversity? Systematist. 2010;**32**:4-8

[10] Ryder OA. Species conservation and systematics: The dilemma of subspecies. Trends in Ecology and Evolution. 1986;**1**:9-10. DOI: 10.1016/0169-5347(86)90059-5

[11] Moritz C. Defining 'evolutionarily significant units' for conservation. Trends in Ecology and Evolution. 1994;**9**:373-375. DOI: 10.1111/j.1365-294X.1994.tb00080.x

[12] Waples RS. Pacific salmon, *Oncorhynchus* spp., and the definition of 'species' under the endangered species act. Marine Fisheries Review. 1991;**53**:11-22

[13] Minh BQ, Klaere S, von Haeseler A. Taxon selection under split diversity. Systematic Biology. 2009;**57**:586-594. DOI: 10.1093/sysbio/syp058

[14] Shapley LS. A value for n-person games. In: Kuhn HW, Tucker AW, editors. Contributions to the Theory of Games. Vol. II. Princeton: Princeton University Press; 1953. pp. 307-317

[15] Steel M, Mimoto A, Mooers AØ. Hedging our bets: The expected contribution of species to future phylogenetic diversity. Evolution Bioinformatic Online. 2007;**3**:237-244

[16] Bottrill MC, Joseph LN, Carwardine J, Bode M, Cook C, et al. Is conservation triage just smart decision making? Trends in Ecology and Evolution. 2008;**23**:649-654. DOI: 10.1016/j.tree.2008.07.007

[17] Igea J, Juste J, Castresana J. Novel intron markers to study the phylogeny of closely related mammalian species. BMC Evolutionary Biology. 2010;**10**:369. DOI: 10.1186/1471-2148-10-369

[18] Fernández-García JL, Díaz Caballero JA, Palacios-González MJ. Linajes mitocondriales del desmán (*Galemys pyrenaicus*) presentes en el LIC "sierra de Gredos y valle del Jerte". Congreso de la SECEM, 4-7 de Diciembre, Burgos, Spain. 2015

[19] Rhymer J, Simberloff D. Extinction by hybridization and introgression. Annual Review of Ecology and Systematics. 1996;**27**:83-109. DOI: 10.1146/annurev.ecolsys.27.1.83

[20] Grant BR, Grant PR. Hybridization and speciation in Darwin's finches: The role of sexual imprinting on a culturally transmitted trait. In: Howard DJ, Berlocher SH, editors. Endless Forms: Species and Speciation. New York: Oxford University Press; 1998. pp. 404-422

[21] Hartl GB, Zachos F, Nadlinger K. Genetic diversity in European red deer (*Cervus elaphus* L.): Anthropogenic influences on natural populations. Comptes Rendus Biologies. 2003;**326**:S37-S42

[22] Fernández-García JL. The endangered *Dama dama mesopotamica*: Genetic variability, allelic loss and hybridization signals. Contributions to Zoology. 2012;**81**(4):223-233

[23] Abbott R, Albach D, Ansell S, Arntzen JW, Baird SJ, Bierne N, Boughman JW, Brelsford A, Buerkle CA, Buggs R, et al. Hybridization and speciation. Journal of Evolutionary Biology. 2013;**26**:229-246. DOI: 10.1111/j.1420-9101.2012.02599.x

[24] Prentis PJ, Wilson JRU, Dormontt EE, Richardson DM, Lowe AJ. Adaptive evolution in invasive species. Trends in Plant Science. 2008;**13**:288-294. DOI: 10.1016/j.tplants.2008.03.004

[25] Seehausen O: Hybridization and adaptive radiation. Trends in Ecology and Evolution. 2004;**19**:198-207. DOI: 10.1016/j.tree.2004.01.003

[26] Grant PR, Grant BR. Phenotypic and genetic effects of hybridization in Darwin's finches. Evolution. 1994;**48**:297-316. DOI: 10.2307/2410094

[27] Kim M, Cui M-L, Cubas P, Gillies A, Lee K, Chapman MA et al. Regulatory genes control a key morphological and ecological trait transferred between species. Science. 2008;**322**:1116-1119. DOI: 10.1126/science.1164371

[28] Arnold ML, Martin NH. Adaptation by introgession. Journal of Biology. 2009;**8**:82. DOI: 10.1186/jbiol176

[29] Whitney KD, Randell RA, Rieseberg LH. Adaptive introgression of abiotic tolerance traits in the sunflower *Helianthus annuus*. New Phytologist. 2010;**187**:230-239. DOI: 10.1111/j.1469-8137.2010.03234.x

[30] Kunte K, Shea C, Aardema ML, Scriber JM, Juenger TE, Gilbert LE, et al. Sex chromosome mosaicism and hybrid speciation among tiger swallowtail butterflies. PLoS Genetics. 2011;**7**:e1002274. DOI: 10.1371/journal.pgen.1002274

[31] Coyne JA, Orr HA. Speciation. Sunderland: Sinauer Associates; 2004. p. 545

[32] Sobel JM, Chen GF, Watt LR, Schemske DW. The biology of speciation. Evolution. 2010;**64**:295-315. DOI: 10.1111/j.1558-5646.2009.00877.x

[33] Servedio MR, Van Doorn GS, Kopp M, Frame AM, Nosil P. Magic traits in speciation: 'Magic' but not rare? Trends in Ecology and Evolution. 2011;**26**:389-397. DOI: 10.1016/j.tree.2011.04.005

[34] Price TD, Bouvier MM. The evolution of F1 postzygotic incompatibilities in birds. Evolution. 2002;**56**:2083-2089

[35] Gourbière S, Mallet J. Are species real? The shape of the species boundary with exponential failure, reinforcement, and the "missing snowball". Evolution. 2010;**64**:1-24. DOI: 10.1111/j.1558-5646.2009.00844.x

[36] Frankham R, Bradshaw CJA, Brook BW. Genetics in conservation management: Revised recommendations for the 50/500 rules, Red List criteria and population viability analyses. Biological Conservation. 2014;**170**:56-63. DOI:10.1016/j.biocon.2013.12.036

[37] Bininda-Emonds O, Vazquez D, Manne L. The calculus of biodiversity: Integrating phylogeny and conservation. Trends in Ecology & Evolution. 2000;**15**(3):92-94

[38] Gaston KJ, Spicer JI. Biodiversity: An Introduction. 2nd edition. Malden: Wiley-Blackwell Publishing; 2004. p. 208

[39] May RM. Taxonomy as destiny. Nature. 1990;**347**:129-130. DOI: 10.1038/347129a0

[40] Faith DP. Conservation evaluation and phylogenetic diversity. Biological Conservation. 1992;**61**:1-10

[41] Pardi F, Goldman N. Species choice for comparative genomics: Being greedy works. PLoS Genetics. 2005;**1**:e71. DOI: 10.1371/journal.pgen.0010071

[42] Marko PB, Hart MW. The complex analytical landscape of gene flow inference. Trends in Ecology and Evolution. 2011;**26**:448-456. DOI: 10.1016/j.tree.2011.05.007

Chapter 3

Phylogenetics, Reticulation and Evolution

Milton H. Gallardo

Additional information is available at the end of the chapter

http://dx.doi.org/10.5772/intechopen.68564

Abstract

Incongruence between phylogenetic trees constructed from different gene sequences has bothered practitioners for decades. Paraphyletic or polyphyletic clustering has been traditionally treated as noise that distorts its genealogical bases. Nevertheless, recent genomic data have provided a first indication that horizontal gene transfer (HGT) in microbes and interspecific hybridization (or polyploidization) in eukaryotes challenge the doctrine of common descent. Due to promiscuous recombination, the initial stages of life would have not had a genealogical history but a common physical one whose graphic representation is known as evolutionary reticulation. Reticulate evolution in plants has long been recognized, and recent genomic evidence from animals also indicates its widespread occurrence. Taking into consideration that mounting evidence for hybridization and polyploidy in eukaryotic taxa accumulates, it is essential to have methods to infer reticulate evolutionary histories. Considering the different forms of transpecific genetic transference and introgression across the tree of life, the origin of a given species may not coincide with the origin of its genes. Accordingly, molecular mutation rates might be erroneous if based on strict genealogical thinking. Given abundant new data, it is time to move forward because a major shift in our understanding of species, speciation and phylogenetics is taking place.

Keywords: convergence, gene trees, phylogenetic incongruence, polyphyly, reticulation

1. Introduction

Since Darwin´s seminal work, it has been claimed that organic diversity could be represented by a unique branching pattern of inclusive hierarchies depicting genealogical relationships among organisms [1]. This tree of life, based on shared homologies, was considered to reflect nature´s genuine attributes, exclusively represented by descent with modification.

Nevertheless, there is neither *a priori* independent evidence nor rigorous tests to ensure such a nested organization of nature's biodiversity due to common descent [2]. In fact, the initial stages of life, including the origin of the last cellular ancestor, were dominated by lateral gene transfer, advanced almost 20 years ago [3]. This breakthrough has challenged the doctrine of common descent by indicating that the ancestral state would not have been an individual but a community of entities with a common physical history, but not with a genealogical one. Apparently, the three domains of life emerged independently through a sorting process from a pool of entities involved in promiscuous recombination. These processes of gene recombination in prokaryotes, leading to reticulate evolution are mimicked by repeated intercrossing (hybridization) between metazoan populations or lineages. Consequently, their evolutionary histories cannot be adequately represented as bifurcating phylogenetic trees. As a result from these deviations, a network of relationships difficult to deal with is produced, regardless of the numerous methods for the reconstruction proposed recently [4].

Traditional phylogenetic analysis applied to animal and plant phyla has stumbled with gross, irreconcilable discrepancies since its onset. Molecular phylogenomics has corrected some of these paradoxes, but what gets clarified on one end gets muddled in another. A paradigmatic example of this is the recent synthesis of animal phylogeny and taxonomy of [5], plagued with conflicts near the base of *Eukaryota* and *Metazoa*. Likewise, the phylogenomic approach to animal evolution by Telford et al. [6] resolved the most derived branches but is contentious with regard to the placement of *Eumetazoa, Bilateria, Protostomia, Deuterostomia* and *Lophotrochozo*a. Likewise, the phylogenetic origin of major plant taxa is unclear. For example, the placement of the Celastrales-Oxalidales-Malpighiales clade within Rosidae remains one of the most confounding phylogenetic questions in angiosperms, with previous analyses placing it with either Fabidae or Malvidae [7].

Theoretically, species correspond to independent, reproductively isolated populations although Darwin recognized interspecific hybridization as a merging process involving two ancestors. The graphical representation of this phenomenon, otherwise being diverging, is known as reticulate evolution or network evolution, describes the origination of a lineage through the partial merging of two ancestor lineages. Hybridization has played an important role in genome diversification and in adapting organisms to their environment. Nevertheless, methods for reconstructing their reticulate relationships are still in their infancy and have limited applicability. Reticulate evolution in plants has long been recognized, but recent genomic evidence from animals indicates that this phenomenon is much more common than anticipated. Taking into consideration that mounting evidence of hybridization in eukaryotic taxa accumulates, it is essential to have methods to infer reticulate evolutionary histories. Given abundant new data, it is time to move forward because a major shift in our understanding of species, speciation and phylogenetics is taking place.

Many groups of closely related species including insects, vertebrates, microbes and plants have reticulate phylogenies. In microbes, lateral gene transfer is the dominant process that distorts strictly genealogical, tree-like phylogenies. In multicellular eukaryotes, hybridization and introgression among related species are of prime importance. Introgression and reticulation can thereby affect all parts of the tree of life, not just the crown species. Accordingly, conceptual issues regarding adaptive evolution, speciation, phylogenetics and comparative genomics must be modified to fit these recent findings. Reticulation is produced by phenomena like lateral gene transfer, introgressive hybridization and polyploidization. In fact, certain alleles of gene trees may appear more closely related to alleles from a different species than to other conspecific alleles, thus giving rise to instances of paraphyly or polyphyly. The occurrence of such anomalous clustering in the evolutionary history of species poses serious challenges to practitioners of phylogenetic analysis as they result in genomic regions with locally incongruent genealogies relative to the speciation pattern. Thus, phylogenetic analyses should account for the reticulate component of evolution, especially now that whole genome sequencing provides unprecedented phylogenetic information across the web of life [8]. Here, we present genetic and genomic evidence indicating the evolutionary importance of reticulation in multicellular eukaryotes and summarize relevant reticulate issues and its bearings on phylogenetic practice.

2. Horizontal gene transfer (HGT)

HGT phenomenon of genetic transference mainly among prokaryotes can occur via bacterial transformation, conjugation or transduction. It excludes mitosis and meiosis and does not require immediate ancestry. Bacterial genomes have revealed a complex evolutionary history, which cannot be represented by a single strictly bifurcating tree for most genes. Comparative analysis of sequenced genomes indicates that lineage-specific gene loss has been common in evolution, thus complicating the notion of a species tree, of a last universal common ancestor and the delimitation of its taxonomic units by being asexual.

HGT in eukaryotes has been reported in phagotrophic protists and limited largely to the ancient acquisition of bacterial genes. Nevertheless, standard mitochondrial genes, encoding ribosomal and respiratory proteins, are subject to evolutionarily frequent horizontal transfer between distantly related flowering plants. These transfers have created a variety of genomic outcomes, including gene duplication, recapture of gene lost through transfer to the nucleus and chimeric, half-monocot, half-dicot genes [9].

As a result, from intergenomic comparisons, HGT appears as a dominant process to generate innovations and complex adaptations like the acquisition of shade-dwelling habits in ferns. Molecular evidence indicates that the chimeric photoreceptor, neochrome, was acquired from hornworts, thereby optimizing phototropic responses [10]. HGT not only involve individual genes but also whole chromosomes and even nuclear genomes by asexual means. In the fungi genus *Fusarium*, HGT was responsible for the acquisition of chromosomes that largely increased the organism pathogenicity [11].

The horizontal transfer of a complete genome, giving rise to a new *Nicotiana* species, was achieved by grafting somatic tissues of two transgenic, 48-chromosome *Nicotiana tabacum* × *Nicotiana glauca*. The resulting octoploid species, *Nicotianu tubauca* ($2n = 96$), has double genome size, and its fertile F1 depicts intermediate phenotypic traits between both parental species [12]. In *Amborella trichopoda* (the sister group of angiosperms), whole mitochondrial transfer and subsequent fusion with the recipient genome have been reported. The plant's huge mitochondrial (mt) genome size (3.9 Mb) comes from six different genomic sources and from the mtDNA of three types of green algae, a fungus and other angiosperms. These findings emphasize the role of transpecific genomic compatibilities, fusions and syngamy, to form more complex wholes [13].

Overall results of reticulate evolution via genome-wide quantification reveal that ecological specialization somehow restricts intra- and interspecific recombination [14]. Nevertheless, the genomic architecture and content of transposable elements are also central to HGT and to recombination potential. In addition, genomic regions differ in levels of potential HGT and reticulated evolution from single genes to whole genomes. It is also noticed that genetic distances, genomic rearrangements and genome synteny all show evidence of HGT and network-like evolution both at whole and core genome scales. Moreover, proteomic core genes have experienced reticulated evolution of complex traits and played a transcendent causal role in the radiation and adaptation of life on earth.

3. Interspecific hybridization

One potential cause of gene tree/species tree discordance and concomitant polyphyly is the occasional mating (hybridization) between otherwise distinct species. The resulting transfer of parental alleles to hybrid offspring (introgression) introduces variation at rates much higher than mutation.

Thus, significant levels of genomic replacement may accrue over long periods, even at low hybridization rates. This has been recently demonstrated in extant *Anopheles* mosquitoes [15] and in some *Heliconius* butterfly species and to detect past hybridization events using ancient DNA [16]. These instances force us to accept an *ad hoc* species definition applicable only to terminal taxa, rather than to the original bifurcating ancestors. Indeed, the branches of the tree change the species identity. Thereby the accumulation of introgressed regions flips the effect of gene majority to another topology [4].

Hybridization is increasingly being recognized as a widespread process between ecologically and behaviorally divergent animal species. Determining phylogenetic relationships in the presence of hybridization remains a major challenge for evolutionary biologists. If hybridization has occurred among the species of a given taxon, cladistic analysis fails to account for the process involved since the relationships are not genealogical but reticulate. Since hybridization results in incongruent intersecting data that obscure the underlying hierarchy, the results are always plagued with convergences and parallelisms of no biological relevancy [17].

Recombination is a form of reticulation that mimics the problems derived from hybridization, except that occurs at the gene level. Recombination can be diagnosed by looking at the compatibility of the phylogenetic partition supported by the polymorphic sites along the sequence. One strategy consists of looking at changes in the most parsimonious topology along sequences, while others use a maximum chi-square test or use the maximum-likelihood approach to detect specific incongruent evolutionary patterns. Unfortunately, no general method to place a putative hybrid in the appropriate clade exists.

Introgression (also known as introgressive hybridization or interspecific gene flow) occurs when alleles from one species penetrate the gene pool of another through interspecific mating and the subsequent backcrossing of hybrids into parental populations. When hybridization is symmetrical, the resulting hybrid species might be polyphyletic, as might be both parental species. Having in mind that hybrid speciation is often associated with whole genome duplication (polyploidy), knowledge of such traits may strengthen the suspicion of polyphyly derived from hybrid speciation [4]. However, in several cases of putative hybrid speciation, alternative explanations have been difficult to rule out. Considering that mitochondrial alleles are more easily introgressed than nuclear ones, their heterospecific plasmidial origin will be more frequently detected. Consequently, mitochondrial gene trees could be particularly susceptible to the effects of introgression and be especially misleading in cases where introgressed haplotype lineages become fixed, leaving no hint that they are of heterospecific origin.

The discovery of cytoplasmic introgression and the disparity between rDNA and cpDNA phylogenies of several plant groups is reflective of past hybridization and subsequent introgression. If an analysis includes hybrids, no matter where the hybrids are placed, a cladistic method produces only divergently branching phylogenetic patterns and thus can never retrieve the correct phylogeny, and we end up with confusing and conflicting results.

4. Polyploidy

Polyploidy is a form of interspecific hybridization followed by whole genome duplication (WGD). As the most drastic modification that a cell can experience, it involves rapid and profound nonrandom changes in chromatin composition, segregation patterns and copy number variation of dispersed repetitive DNA [18, 19]. Polyploidy is also instrumental to introgress alien DNA into breeding lines enabling the introduction of novel characters as demonstrated by FISH, GISH and genetic mapping [20]. Its evolutionary role has motivated intense studies because duplicated gene pathways provide new opportunities for increased body-plan complexity, organismal differentiation and adaptation by recruitment of new genes to new roles [21, 22]. Polyploidy has played a significant role in the hybrid speciation and adaptive radiation of flowering plants but has been considered irrelevant to mammalian speciation due to severe disruptions in the sex-determination system and dosage compensation mechanism [23, 24]. Recent comparative genomic data has further demonstrated the evolutionary transcendence of polyploidy by reporting three rounds of WGD (3R hypothesis) in vertebrate evolution [25] and five rounds in flowering plants [26].

The convergence of distinct lineages upon interspecific hybridization (allopolyploid) and subsequent endoreduplication that increases ploidy level is a driving force in the origin of most flowering plants species. Likewise, the grass tribe *Triticeae* (Hordeeae) is characterized by its evolutionary complexity as indicated by numerous events of auto- and allopolyploidization. Introgression involving diploid and polyploid ancestors is the major factor concurring to their complex history [27]. Moreover, several analyses of multi-gene data sets demonstrated the conflict between the chloroplast and both nuclear and mitochondrial data sets. Nevertheless, synthetic polyploids are able to stabilize their genome in few generations after their onset.

In order to explain conflicting pattern distribution in a phylogeny, it is claimed that several strategies have been advanced [7].

Following WGD, duplicated genes show two types of homologies stem from the fact that genes are duplicated: paralogy and orthology. Paralogy stands for genes that are related following a duplication event, whereas orthology is the result of speciation. Consequently, the gene tree based on multigene families in polyploid species would be problematic if confounding these two forms of homology. Due to this limitation, mitochondrial single-copy genes rather than nuclear genes are a more reliable source of allele orthology. A gene tree that includes paralogous alleles may depict polyphyletic species because its topology reflects gene duplication as well as speciation. The cause of this polyphyly may be misinterpreted if the orthology of alleles is assumed. Because mitochondrial loci are single-copy genes rather than members of multigene families, it was long considered safe to assume allele orthology by mitochondrial primers. This is a serious phylogenetic challenge considering that most angiosperms are polyploid. If the 3R and 5R hypotheses are scientifically valid, their implication makes the search for common ancestry irrelevant to science. To celebrate the 150 years of Darwin´s Origin of Species, the prestigious journal, *Heredity*, published an issue on speciation whose editorial introduction says: "many questions concerning the causes of speciation remain open and speciation continues to be one of the most actively studied topics in modern evolutionary biology" [28]. The end result is that we neither do have a comprehensive understanding of speciation nor about the reality of the species. And the origin of species by natural selection continues being debated. One wonders whether the scientific community is not pursuing in the wrong direction by studying patterns instead of the process itself [1, 3]. In this line, Lynn Margulis claimed that "...neodarwinism will ultimately be viewed as only a minor twentieth-century religious sect within the sprawling religious persuasion of Anglo-Saxon biology" [29].

In short, gene duplication following polyploidy can give rise to multigenic families that correspond to groups of locally distributed, tandemly oriented redundant genes that can subsequently be involved in non-allelic homologous recombination. Duplicated genes can undergo three different outcomes. First, both copies can persist, keeping their sequence identity while maintaining a high level of gene expression. A second possibility, known as subfunctionalization, occurs when one gene copy is silenced (by physical elimination or methylation). Subfunctionalized copies may form pseudogenes, nonfunctional genetic sequences that conserve their similarity to one or more paralogs that confound phylogenetic analyses. The third outcome of a duplicated gene is neofunctionalization, a phenomenon that involves functional diversification to a new role or allelic specialization of a previous function. Clearly, these processes of gene evolution consisting of both gene births and deaths after duplication interfere with the general assumptions of phylogenetic analysis and blur the end results.

5. Incomplete lineage sorting

Incomplete lineage sorting occurs when polymorphisms persist between speciation events, so that the true genealogical relationship of a gene or genome region differs from the species branching pattern. Incomplete lineage sorting and introgression are two main causes of discordance between gene trees and species trees of eukaryotic coding sequences. For instance, around 15% of human genes are more closely related to homologs in gorillas than to the chimpanzee sister lineage. This anomaly is probably derived from their reduced ancestral effective population size (N_e) and short speciation time span between humans and simians. Recent findings of shared polymorphisms between them include the MHC and ABO blood group loci. In the species complex of *Anopheles gambiae*, a very large chromosomal inversion encompassing 8.5% of its genome size is maintained by a balanced selection-driven populational regime [15]. Unlike lateral transfer and introgression, incomplete lineage sorting does not result in phylogenetic reticulation at species level. Nevertheless, it confounds molecular phylogenetic analysis by making to appear closer that real two different clades. A phenomenon derived from chance events is taken as if genealogical.

Several analytical methods assume that reticulation events are the sole cause of all incongruence among the gene trees and seek phylogenetic networks to explain all incongruences. Nevertheless, these methods overestimate the degree of reticulation if other causes of incongruence are at play. Indeed, recent studies in the human genome [30, 31] in *Mus* [32] and butterflies [33] have shown that detecting hybridization in practice is complicated by incomplete lineage sorting.

Some authors claim that significant steps have been conducted to put phylogenetic networks on par with phylogenetic trees as a model of capturing evolutionary relationships. Nevertheless, progress with phylogenetic network inference notwithstanding methods of inferring reticulate evolutionary histories while accounting for ILS is poorly understood. Its inapplicability stems mainly from two major issues: the lack of a phylogenetic network inference method and the lack of a method to assess the degree of confidence associated to an inference traveling into a phylogenetic network space. Likewise, methods for assessing the complexity of a network and the use the bootstrap method for measuring branch support of inferred networks have been developed [33].

6. Identifying complex patterns of genetic diversity through networks

Branching diagrams dominate the phylogenetic thinking. Nevertheless, the genetic patterns of bacterial genome evolution give rise to complex patterns than cannot be accommodated by a tree [34]. The complexity and profound relationships among the three domains of life defy traditional methods. For example, the construction of a web of genetic similarity comprising proteomic data from 14 eukaryotes, 104 prokaryotes, 2389 virus and 1044 plasmids clearly showed the chimeric origin of eukaryotes. These fusion events between *Archaebacteria* and *Eubacteria* would not have been detected by conventional phylogenetic algorithms and trees. But not only that, it also indicated that eukaryote genes connecting a specified domain of prokaryotes tend to connect to other entities of the same domain [35]. Genes derived from *Archaea* or *Bacteria* tend to carry out different functions and act in distinct cell compartments. This complex interwoven on the web suggests an early integration of their respective genetic repertoires. Thus, web analysis stresses the study of deep evolutionary events.

Reticulate patterns can also stem from an inadequate analysis or data processing, wrong specification of the model used, wrong use of data or sequence alignments. Even though network analysis allows a drastic reduction of data misinterpretation, most important is to be aware that genomic hybridization is a more probable explanation to capture the differences among genetic trees [36].

7. Conclusions

Interspecific gene exchanges are much common than previously appreciated. This not only includes hybridizing sister species undergoing genomic introgression but whole groups that exchange adaptive and nonadaptive genomic regions, as exemplified in *Anopheles, Heliconius* and hominids. Considering that hybridization between sister species may or may not affect the species tree, the sole estimates of introgression rates derived from species tree topologies can underestimate the overall level of gene flow. Thus, the origin of traits and the genes behind them can have very different histories from that of the species tree.

The only literature survey dealing with the frequency, causes and consequences of species-level paraphyly and polyphyly indicates that their incidence is taxonomically widespread [37]. Interestingly, almost 25% of the scientific literature surveyed does not offer an explanation to polyphyletic gene trees. Polyphyly was observed in 15% of species across the cnidarians, mollusks, insects, crustaceans, arachnids and echinoderms, whereas half of the citations dealing with these deviations claim for a faulty taxonomy. Both introgressive hybridization and incomplete lineage sorting were also invoked in one third of the 2319 species analysed. Inadequate phylogenetic information is invoked in few papers [37]. Consequently, species-level monophyly cannot be assumed as an *a priori* axiom. For the origination of above species-level polyphyly, traditional phylogenetics uses a Lamarckian explanation and thinking: the environment triggers evolutionary innovations, while organisms passively adapt to the new environmental demands. Natural selection is conceived as the source and driving force that shape life as we see it. Distance and objectivity of phylogenetic thinking from a particular (i.e. Darwinian) evolutionary view is advised. The search for evolutionary relationships does not require alignment to a particular world view to discover the pattern that connects [38]. Otherwise, any data set that does not fit the model is labelled as convergence or parallelism, descriptive concepts with no informational, explanatory value. The morphophysiological discrepancies observed among animal or vegetal phyla [5–7] are incontrovertible evidence that traditional phylogenetic thinking cannot explain the origin of body plans. Distorted presumptions about nature and inadequate or faulty methodologies conspire to maintain the present phylogenetic incongruencies. Having in mind that HGT occurs all across the tree of life, the time for the origin of a given species will not coincide with the origin of its genes. They could have evolved in other genetic backgrounds and horizontally transferred across reproductive barriers. Accordingly, molecular mutation rates might be erroneous if based on genealogical thinking. One explanation for polyphyly might not be derived from a faulty taxonomy but from unforeseen non-Mendelian mechanisms.

Acknowledgements

The assistance of E. Suárez-Villota is highly appreciated. This contribution was supported with private funds.

Author details

Milton H. Gallardo

Address all correspondence to: mgallard@uach.cl

Faculty of Sciences, Institute of Marine and Limnological Sciences, Austral University of Chile, Valdivia, Chile

References

[1] Woese CR. A new biology for a new century. Microbiology and Molecular Biology Reviews. 2004;**68**:173-186. DOI: 10.1128/MMBR.68.2.173-186.2004

[2] Puigbo P, Lobkovsky AE, Kristensen DM, Wolf YI, Koonin EV. Genomes in turmoil: Quantification of genome dynamics in prokaryote supergenomes. BMC Biology. 2014;**12**:66. DOI: 10.1186/s12915-014-0066-4

[3] Woese CR. The universal ancestor. Proceedings of the National Academy of Sciences. 1998;**95**:6854-6859. DOI: 10.1073/pnas.95.12.6854

[4] Mallet J, Besansky N, Hahn MW. How reticulated are species? Bioessays. 2016;**38**:140-149. DOI: 10.1002/bies.201500149

[5] Hinchliff CE, Smith SA, Allman JF, Burleigh JG, Chaudhary R, Coghill LM, Crandall KA, Deng J, Drew BT, Gazis R, et al. Synthesis of phylogeny and taxonomy into a comprehensive tree of life. Proceedings of the National Academy of Sciences. 2015;**112**:12764-12769. DOI: 10.1073/pnas.1423041112

[6] Telford MJ, Budd Graham E, Philippe H. Phylogenomic Insights into animal evolution. Current Biology. 2015;**25**:R876-R887. DOI: 10.1016/j.cub.2015.07.060

[7] Sun M, Soltis DE, Soltis PS, Zhu X, Burleigh JG, Chen Z. Deep phylogenetic incongruence in the angiosperm clade *Rosidae*. Molecular Phylogenetics and Evolution. 2015;**83**:156-166. DOI: 10.1016/j.ympev.2014.11.003

[8] Corel E, Lopez P, Meheust R, Bapteste E. Network-thinking: Graphs to analyze microbial complexity and evolution. Trends in Microbiology. 2016;**24**:224-237. DOI: 10.1016/j.tim.2015.12.003

[9] Bergthorsson U, Adams KL, Thomason B, Palmer JD. Widespread horizontal transfer of mitochondrial genes in flowering plants. Nature. 2003;**424**:197-201. DOI: 10.1038/nature01743

[10] Li FW, Villarreal JC, Kelly S, Rothfels CJ, Melkonian M, Frangedakis E, Ruhsam M, Sigel EM, Der JP, Pittermann J, et al. Horizontal transfer of an adaptive chimeric photoreceptor from bryophytes to ferns. Proceedings of the National Academy of Sciences of the United States of America. 2014;**111**:6672-6677. DOI: 10.1073/pnas.1319929111

[11] Mehrabi R, Bahkali AH, Abd-Elsalam KA, Moslem M, Ben M'barek S, Gohari AM, Jashni MK, Stergiopoulos I, Kema GH, de Wit PJ. Horizontal gene and chromosome transfer in plant pathogenic fungi affecting host range. FEMS Microbiology Reviews. 2011;**35**:542-554. DOI: 10.1111/j.1574-6976.2010.00263.x

[12] Fuentes I, Stegemann S, Golczyk H, Karcher D, Bock R. Horizontal genome transfer as an asexual path to the formation of new species. Nature. 2014;**511**:232-235. DOI: 10.1038/nature13291

[13] Rice DW, Alverson AJ, Richardson AO, Young GJ, Sanchez-Puerta MV, Munzinger J, Barry K, Boore JL, Zhang Y, dePamphilis CW, et al. Horizontal transfer of entire genomes via mitochondrial fusion in the angiosperm *Amborella*. Science. 2013;**342**:1468-1473. DOI: 10.1126/science.1246275

[14] Hernández-López A, Chabrol O, Royer-Carenzi M, Merhej V, Pontarotti P, Raoult D. To tree or not to tree? Genome-wide quantification of recombination and reticulate evolution during the diversification of strict intracellular bacteria. Genome Biology and Evolution. 2013;**5**:2305-2317. DOI: 10.1093/gbe/evt178

[15] Wen D, Yu Y, Hahn MW, Nakhleh L. Reticulate evolutionary history and extensive introgression in mosquito species revealed by phylogenetic network analysis. Molecular Ecology. 2016;**25**:2361-2372. DOI: 10.1111/mec.13544

[16] Schaefer NK, Shapiro B, Green RE. Detecting hybridization using ancient DNA. Molecular Ecology. 2016;**25**:2398-2412. DOI: 10.1111/mec.13556

[17] Funk VA. Phylogenetic patterns and hybridization. Annals of the Missouri Botanical Garden. 1985;**66**(3):521-527. DOI: 10.2307/2399220

[18] Chen ZJ. Genetic and epigenetic mechanisms for gene expression and phenotypic variation in plant polyploids. Annual Review of Plant Biology. 2007;**58**:377-406. DOI: 10.1146/annurev.arplant.58.032806.103835

[19] Lim KY, Soltis DE, Soltis PS, Tate J, Matyasek R, Srubarova H, Kovarik A, Pires JC, Xiong Z, Leitch AR. Rapid chromosome evolution in recently formed polyploids in *Tragopogon* (Asteraceae). PLoS One. 2008;**3**:e3353. DOI: 10.1371/journal.pone.0003353

[20] Chester M, Leitch AR, Soltis PS, Soltis DE. Review of the application of modern cytogenetic methods (FISH/GISH) to the study of reticulation (polyploidy/hybridisation). Genes. 2010;**1**:166-192. DOI: 10.3390/genes1020166

[21] Otto SP. The evolutionary consequences of polyploidy. Cell. 2007;**131**:452-462. DOI: 10.1016/j.cell.2007.10.022

[22] Otto SP, Whitton J. Polyploid incidence and evolution. Annual Review of Genetics. 2000;**34**:401-437. DOI: 10.1146/annurev.genet.34.1.401

[23] Gallardo MH, Gonzalez CA, Cebrian I. Molecular cytogenetics and allotetraploidy in the red vizcacha rat, *Tympanoctomys barrerae* (*Rodentia, Octodontidae*). Genomics. 2006;**88**:214-221. DOI: 10.1016/j.ygeno.2006.02.010

[24] Suárez-Villota EY, Vargas RA, Marchant CL, Torres JE, Kohler N, Nunez JJ, de la Fuente R, Page J, Gallardo MH. Distribution of repetitive DNAs and the hybrid origin of the red vizcacha rat (*Octodontidae*). Genome. 2012;**55**:105-117. DOI: 10.1139/G11-084

[25] Pascual-Anaya J, D'Aniello S, Kuratani S, Garcia-Fernandez J. Evolution of *Hox* gene clusters in Deuterostomes. BMC Developmental Biology. 2013;**13**:26. DOI: 10.1186/1471-213X-13-26

[26] Jiao Y, Wickett NJ, Ayyampalayam S, Chanderbali AS, Landherr L, Ralph PE, Tomsho LP, Hu Y, Liang H, Soltis PS, et al. Ancestral polyploidy in seed plants and angiosperms. Nature. 2011;**473**:97-100. DOI: 10.1038/nature09916

[27] Mason-Gamer RJ. Phylogeny of a genomically diverse group of *Elymus* (*Poaceae*) allopolyploids reveals multiple levels of reticulation. PLoS One. 2013;**8**:e78449. DOI: 10.1371/journal.pone.0078449

[28] Butlin RK, Ritchie MG. Genetics of speciation. Heredity. 2009;**102**:1-3. DOI: 10.1038/hdy.2008.97

[29] Mann C. Lynn Margulis: Science's unruly earth mother. Science. 1991;**252**:378-381. DOI: 10.1126/science.252.5004.378

[30] Eriksson A, Manica A. Effect of ancient population structure on the degree of polymorphism shared between modern human populations and ancient hominins. Proceedings of the National Academy of Sciences of the United States of America. 2012;**109**:13956-13960. DOI: 10.1073/pnas.1200567109

[31] Green RE, Krause J, Briggs AW, Maricic T, Stenzel U, Kircher M, Patterson N, Li H, Zhai W, Fritz MH-Y, et al. A draft sequence of the Neandertal Genome. Science. 2010;**328**:710. DOI: 10.1126/science.1188021

[32] Staubach F, Lorenc A, Messer PW, Tang K, Petrov DA, Tautz D. Genome patterns of selection and introgression of haplotypes in natural populations of the house mouse (*Mus musculus*). PLoS Genetics. 2012;**8**:e1002891. DOI: 10.1371/journal.pgen.1002891

[33] Moody ML, Rieseberg LH. Sorting through the chaff, nDNA gene trees for phylogenetic inference and hybrid identification of annual sunflowers (*Helianthus* sect. *Helianthus*). Molecular Phylogenetics and Evolution. 2012;**64**:145-155. DOI: dx.doi.org/10.1016/j.ympev.2012.03.012

[34] Jachiet PA, Colson P, Lopez P, Bapteste E. Extensive gene remodeling in the viral world: New evidence for nongradual evolution in the mobilome network. Genome Biology and Evolution. 2014;**6**:2195-2205. DOI: 10.1093/gbe/evu168

[35] Alvarez-Ponce D, Lopez P, Bapteste E, McInerney JO. Gene similarity networks provide tools for understanding eukaryote origins and evolution. Proceedings of the National Academy of Sciences of the United States of America. 2013;**110**:E1594-E1603. DOI: 10.1073/pnas.1211371110

[36] Bapteste E, van Iersel L, Janke A, Kelchner S, Kelk S, McInerney JO, Morrison DA, Nakhleh L, Steel M, Stougie L, Whitfield J. Networks: Expanding evolutionary thinking. Trends in Genetics. 2013;**29**:439-441. DOI: 10.1016/j.tig.2013.05.007

[37] Funk DJ, Omland KE. Species-level paraphyly and polyphyly: Frequency, causes, and consequences, with insights from animal mitochondrial DNA. Annual Review of Ecology, Evolution, and Systematics. 2003;**34**:397-423. DOI: 10.1146/annurev.ecolsys.34.011802.132421

[38] Bateson G. Mind and Nature. A Necessary Unity. New York: Bantam Books; 1979. p. 259

Section 2

Cytogenetics and Genomics Approaches for Phylogenetics

Chapter 4

Applying Cytogenetics in Phylogenetic Studies

Ming Chen, Wen-Hsiang Lin, Dong-Jay Lee,
Shun-Ping Chang, Tze-Ho Chen and Gwo-Chin Ma

Additional information is available at the end of the chapter

http://dx.doi.org/10.5772/intechopen.68566

Abstract

Cytogenetics, with its fundamental role in the field of genetic investigation, continues to be an indispensable tool for studying phylogenetics, given that currently molecular evolutionary analyses are more commonly utilized. Chromosomal evolution indicated that genomic evolution occurs at the level of chromosomal segments, namely, the genomic blocks in the size of Mb-level. The recombination of homologous blocks, through the mechanisms of insertion, translocation, inversion, and breakage, has been proven to be a major mechanism of speciation and subspecies differentiation. Meanwhile, molecular cytogenetics (fluorescence in situ hybridization-based methodologies) had been already widely applied in studying plant genetics since polyploidy is common in plant evolution and speciation. It is now recognized that comparative cytogenetic studies can be used to explore the plausible phylogenetic relationships of the extant mammalian species by reconstructing the ancestral karyotypes of certain lineages. Therefore, cytogenetics remains a feasible tool in the study of comparative genomics, even in this next generation sequencing (NGS) prevalent era.

Keywords: cytogenetics, comparative cytogenetics, fluorescence *in situ* hybridization, genomic *in situ* hybridization, zoo-CGH

1. Introduction: chromosomal evolution of mammals

According to fossil records, the radiation evolution of mammals diverged after the K-T boundary (approximately 65 Mya, between the Cretaceous and Tertiary periods, at which most of the dinosaurs were extinct). There are three hypotheses that try to explain such findings: (1) Explosive hypothesis: It is supported by most paleobiologists and states that the genesis and diversification of many phyletic groups ("Orders") diverged after the Cretaceous-Tertiary (K-T) boundary; (2) Long Fuse hypothesis: It supports the view that Order diversification occurred after the K-T boundary but that genesis occurred in the Cretaceous period, i.e., before the K-T boundary; and (3) Short Fuse hypothesis: It considers the genesis and diversification of Orders to have diverged before the K-T boundary (**Figure 1**) [1].

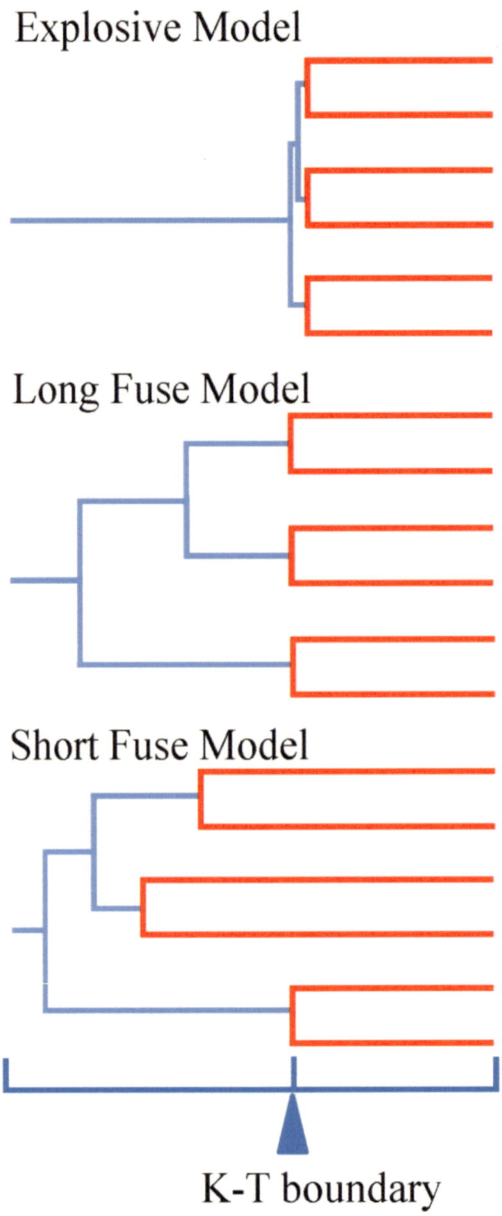

Figure 1. Three hypotheses of mammalian interordinal divergences, modified from Ref. [1].

http://dx.doi.org/10.5772/intechopen.68566

Molecular data indicate that mammalian diversification began in the Cretaceous period, which supports the (2) Long Fuse and (3) Short Fuse hypotheses. However, these data have limitations, including the availability of a single temporal calibration point and the variable evolution rate of different phyletic groups. Due to the lack of representativeness of the samples, this inadequate taxon sampling restricts the use on some, but not all, placental mammals, and it makes the negative correlation between evolution rate and body size difficult to explain. William Murphy and Stephen O'Brien's team made a successful attempt at answering these questions with zoo-fluorescence *in situ* hybridization (zoo-FISH). Currently, the Long Fuse hypothesis seems to be a better match with the evolution of most phyletic groups, but not the orders *Rodentia* and *Eulipotyphla*, which better suit the Short Fuse hypothesis [1].

Figure 2 presents the phylogenetic tree of placental mammals derived from 16,379 nucleotide sequences (including 19 nuclear genes and 3 mitochondrial genes published by the study team), where opossum is considered an outgroup using the maximal likelihood method, and placental mammals are considered to appear at 105 Mya. When the K-T boundary is labeled with red dashes, we find that "Order" genesis and diversification are events that occur before the boundary.

By comparing the chromosomal break point of multiple species, including the chromosomal rearrangement of loci discovered via comparative genomics and some genetic sequences from

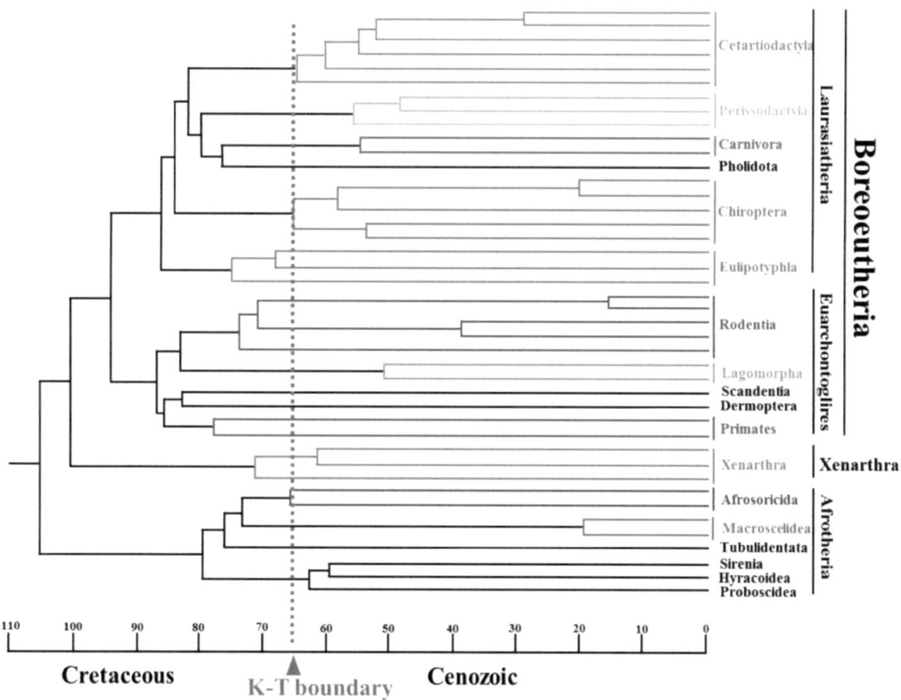

Figure 2. Phylogenetic tree of placental mammals derived from 16,379 nucleotide sequences, modified from Ref. [1].

fully sequenced species, we can clearly find that (1) Approximately 20% of chromosomal break points are repeatedly involved in the evolutionary process of mammals. (2) These repeatedly involved break points are primarily located at the centromere and telomere. (3) The number of genes within and near the break point blocks that are involved in chromosomal evolution is higher than the mean of the overall genome. (4) The unique break points unique in Primates are located at repeated segment regions and the ends are surrounded by reversed sequences. **Figure 3** refers to the rate of chromosomal breaking using the chromosomal break points involved in the evolution of mammals.

The result shows that the chromosomal rearrangement rate before the K-T boundary is 0.11–0.43/My, and this rate is doubled to quadrupled for Primates and increased fivefold for Rodentia [2, 3].

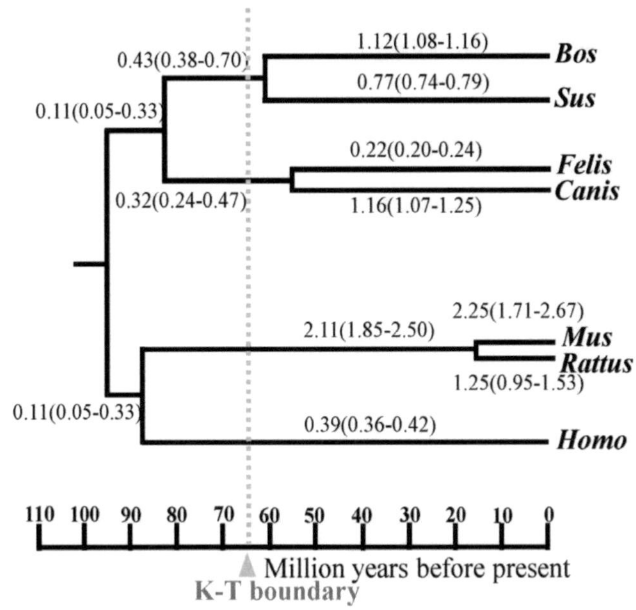

Figure 3. Rate of chromosomal breaking using chromosomal break points involved in the evolution of mammals, modified from Ref. [3].

2. How to apply molecular genomics in the study of evolution and parental relationships

2.1. Zoo-FISH

Comparative mapping: It is a method for comparing the location of homologous genes of different species to explore the evolution of genomes; zoo-FISH is an extension of such technology. This method assesses the overall chromosomal similarity among all mammalian orders and becomes a powerful tool to study genomic evolution. The possible mechanism and factors related to mammalian genomic evolution can be understood with Metatheria and Eutheria studies.

When conducting zoo-FISH, partial or whole chromosomes are obtained through the sorting of fluorescence-labeled cells or microscopic extraction. DNA extracted from this specific chromosomal block is subject to degenerated oligonucleotide primed-PCR (DOP-PCR), then labeled with fluorescence to produce probes, and hybridized with the chromosome of the species of interest. Due to the resolution of zoo-FISH, which is approximately 10 Mbp (megabase pairs), this method may underestimate the real rearrangement events on the chromosome. However, zoo-FISH has revealed some interesting facts: many chromosome blocks of different species are rather conservative, and the similar chromosome blocks from a common ancestor are called synteny blocks. For example, one somatic chromosome of the gray-headed flying fox (*Pteropus poliocephalus*) possesses synteny blocks that are also found in *Homo sapiens* (HSA) chromosome 3 and HSA 21. These HSA3+21 synteny blocks form the primary synteny blocks of placental mammals, i.e., it is a characteristic that was present in a common ancestor and all researched Eutheria members [4].

One of the most important applications of zoo-FISH is to study the speed of chromosomal rearrangement when studying genomic evolution [5]. Using the phylogenetic tree that is based on fossil evidence, we can understand the rate of movement and rearrangement of synteny blocks in the chromosomes of two species. When there are difficulties in bi-directional zoo-FISH, monodirectional zoo-FISH can provide with key information or a new understanding. By comparing the chromosomal synteny blocks of indicator mammals and Aves, the occurrence rate of chromosomal rearrangement was found to be fixed at approximately 1–10/Mya [6]. The chromosomal rearrangement rate is shown in **Figure 4**, and the rate may differ with lineage genesis and at different evolutionary stages.

Three important stages of chromosomal rearrangement are found (**Figure 4**): The first stage (1–3 Mya) < 0.2/My, the second stage increased to 1.1/My, and in the third stage, the rearrangement rate greatly varied in nonrodents. For example, humans, *Carnivora* and *Soricidae* are of low rearrangement (< 0.1/My), swine, cattle, equine and dolphin are moderate (0.1–0.3/My), and large apes are relatively fast (1.5–2.3/My). The chromosomal evolution in Rodentia is the fastest, and the possible explanations include (1) population size (a larger population provides more genetic modification); (2) different genetic composition (more than 50% of the mammalian genome is repeated sequence, whereas it is only 15% repeated sequence in birds), and (3) different generation times (a short generation time indicates more mitotic events). From chromosomal evolutionary evidence, scientists believe that the evolution of mammalian genomes was inconsistent. The evolution was faster for Rodentia, bears, canines, cattle and few big apes, whereas it was relatively slow for cats, ferrets, badgers, dolphins and humans. In addition, it is worth noting that zoo-FISH, like other FISH-based methods, cannot identify intrachromosomal rearrangements (such as inversion). It was believed that the incidence of interchromosomal rearrangement events is higher than intrachromosomal events, but a sequential comparison revealed that it is the opposite for feline and cattle. In a zoo-FISH using human DNA as probe, some recombination events were lineage-specific. For

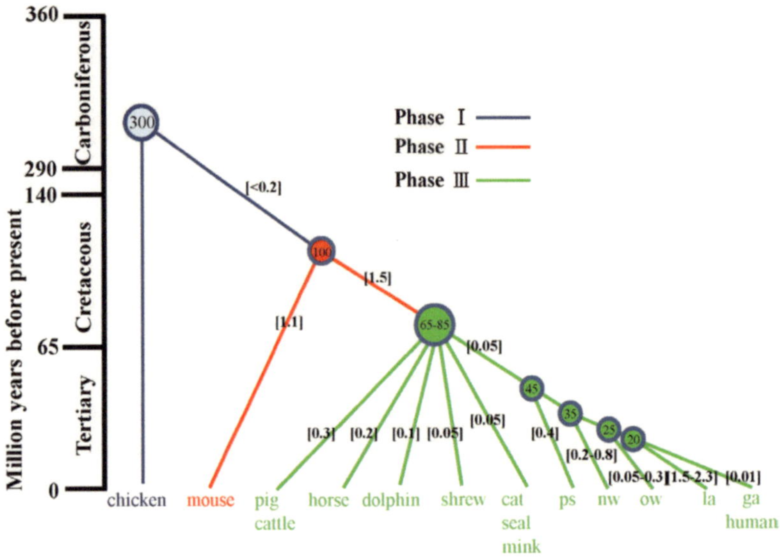

Figure 4. Three phases of chromosomal rearrangement rate. The numbers in the circles are the time (Mya) of divergence of common ancestors, and the numbers in the brackets indicate the rates of chromosomal rearrangement per Myr. (ps= prosimians; nw= new world monkeys; ow = old world monkeys; la = lesser apes; ga = great apes.) Modified from Ref. [6].

example, "15 + 19" (suggesting synteny blocks similar to HSA15 and 19) is Cetartiodactyla- and Perissodactyla-specific, "3 + 19" is Carnivora-specific, and "14 + 15" is widely seen in Aves and placental mammals other than Rodentia (**Figure 5**).

The other application of zoo-FISH is to reconstruct primitive karyotyping. **Figure 6** shows the estimates of ancestral placental mammal ($2n = 50$), primate ($2n = 50$), and Carnivora ($2n = 42$) karyotypes as well as each chromosome and its relationship with human syntenic-associated chromosomes.

It is worth noting that the study shows that the chromosomal karyotype of primitive placental mammals is $2n = 50$, while Svartman et al. [7] also found that the karyotype of Hoffmann's two-toed sloth (*Choloepus hoffmanni*), a Xenarthra member, possesses a karyotype close to the primitive one. This result suggests that the most primitive placental mammals may be Xenarthra, not Afrotheria. Both groups originated in the southern hemisphere, and this result does not violate Murphy's hypothesis on the origin of mammals. That is, when the part of supercontinent Gondwana in southern hemisphere had not yet separated and formed Africa and South America, placental mammals diverged and Xenarthra and Afrotheria appeared; later, the ancestors of Laurasiatheria and Euarchontoglires diverged and migrated to the northern hemisphere.

The karyotype of Hoffmann's two-toed sloth: The blocks that are syntenic to HSA are labeled on the left of each chromosome. For example, Chromosome 1 is syntenic to HSA1, but it is not syntenic to other HSA chromosomes, while Chromosome 6 contains synteny blocks that are similar to those found in HSA3 and HSA21 [7]. These karyotypes are presented in **Figure 7**.

http://dx.doi.org/10.5772/intechopen.68566

Superorder/order	Species	Syntenic block associations																							
		12/22	16/19	14/15	3/21	7/16	4/8p	5/19p	1q/10q	3/19p	10p/12	5/21	18/22	11/19	2/8/4	3/20	18/19	2/8	7/10	4/20	2/20	1/10p	20/15	12/8	10/16
Cetartiodactyla	Dolphin	●	●	●	●	●		●					●												
	Indian muntjac	●	●	●	●	●		●				●	●												
	Pig	●	●	●	●	●	●	●						●											
	Camel	●	●	●	●	●	●	●																	
	Cow	●	●	●	●	●	●	●	●																
Perissodactyla	Rhinoceros	●		●	●	●	●	●	●																
	Zebra	●	●	●	●	●	●	●	●					●											
	Horse	●		●	●	●	●	●	●					●											
Carnivora	Cat	●	●	●	●	●	●			●	●		●								●				
	Dog	●		●	●	●	●		●	●															
	Giant panda	●	●		●		●			●															
Pholldota	Pangolin	●	●	●	●	●	●		●							●			●						
Chiroptera	Bat	●	●	●	●	●	●																		
Eullpotyphla	Shrew hedgehog	●		●	●	●	●				●	●						●		●					
	Common shrew	●	●	●	●	●	●			●										●					
Rodentia	Gray squirrel	●	●	●	●	●	●														●	●	●	●	
Lagomorpha	Rabbit	●	●	●	●	●	●														●	●			
Scandentia	Tree shrew	●	●	●	●																				●
Primates	Howler monkey			●	●				●					●											
	Slow loris	●		●	●	●																			
Xenarthra	Two-toed sloth	●		●	●	●	●											●	●						
	Anteater	●	●	●	●	●	●					●						●	●						
Afrotheria	Aardvark	●	●	●	●	●	●				●	●			●	●									
	African elephant	●	●	●	●	●					●	●					●								
	Golden mole	●	●	●	●	●	●				●	●			●										

Figure 5. Human synteny block associations observed in other placental mammals by zoo-FISH, and positive results were indicated by the solid circles, modified from Ref. [4].

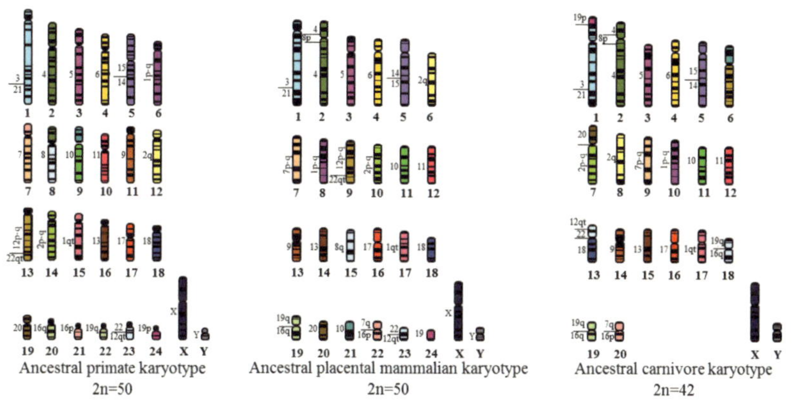

Figure 6. Assumed ancestral karyotypes. Numbers at the left side of the ideogram indicate the regions homologous to human karyotype segments, modified from Ref. [4].

2.2. How is chromosomal recombination fixed in evolution?

Theoretically, chromosomal rearrangement may lead to meiotic errors and reduced fertility. It is fundamentally a harmful genetic variation, and most rearrangements are difficult to pass on in a population. However, (1) genetic drift, (2) Muller's ratchet mechanism or (3) hitch-hiker make it possible to keep some chromosomal recombination (beneficial mutations may be eliminated due to the selection of other loci, whereas harmful mutations may be preserved due to the selection of other beneficial loci).

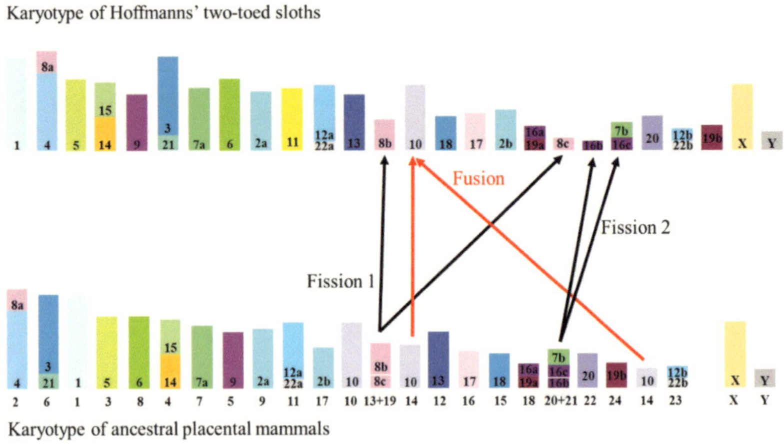

Figure 7. The karyotype of Hoffmann's two-toed sloth is arranged from left to right in the order of chromosomal number, the number in the column refers to the number of HSA it is syntenic to, and the diagram below karyotype of ancestral placental mammals describes the synteny blocks in sloth chromosome. We can find that both are quite similar but one is subject to two fissions and one fusion, modified from Ref. [7].

2.3. The importance of studying "the weird mammals"

The genome of most mammals contains approximately 3 billion nucleotides (3×10^9 bp), but the number of chromosome varies greatly. For placental mammals, Indian muntjac possesses as few as $2n = 6$, while South America rodents possess $2n = 92$; and for opossum, swamp wallaby possesses as few as $2n = 10$, while rufous rat kangaroo possesses $2n = 32$. Long, conservative synteny blocks are found in placental mammals. For example, mice and humans share 116 synteny blocks, and it is estimated that approximately 94 rearrangement events have occurred.

Infraclasses Eutheria (placental mammals) and Metatheria (opossum) diverged at approximately 130 Mya, and their subclasses, Theria and Prototheria (i.e., monotreme), diverged at approximately 170 Mya. Fossil studies show that the radiation evolution of placental mammals (20 orders, including more than 4600 species) occurred in the Cretaceous period (approximately 60–80 Mya). By comparing the differences in the genomes of various animal populations, especially those that play specific roles in evolutionary history (Jennifer Graves, an Australian scholar, called them "the weird mammals"), such as monotreme, opossum and fast-evolving rodents, we can learn more about the evolution progress of mammals.

3. The innovative application of zoological comparative genomic hybridization (CGH) in phylogenetics

Placental mammals include four major lineages: (1) Afrotheria, which includes the orders Sirenia, Hyracoidea, Proboscidea, Tubulidentata, Macroscelidea and Afrosoricida; (2) Laurasiatheria, which includes orders Eulipotyphla, Carnivora, Pholidota, Perissodactyla, Cetartiodactyla and Chiroptera; (3) Euarchontoglires, which includes Rodentia, Lagomorpha, Primates, Scandentia and Dermoptera; and (4) Xenarthra [8]. Currently, there are disputes and uncertainties in the phylogenetic relationships and the true origins of each order in these four lineages. We attempt to define the phylogenetic relationship of the orders Pholidota, Carnivora and Xenarthra using genomic *in situ* hybridization, which was used to determine such relationships for plants. In fact, there is a similar technology called "DNA-DNA hybridization," developed by Sibley and Ahlquist [9]. The basic premise of DNA-DNA hybridization is that a single strand is obtained from the DNA double helix of each species, and when the single strands are hybridized, the binding of the strands from two different species will be much stronger and their associated melting temperatures will be higher when they have a closer relationship. Radioisotope labeling is used to verify the binding as reformation of the double helix or the combination of single strands from two compared species. This technology was applied in the determination of the phylogenetic relationship between Primates and Aves. This technology revealed that in hominoids, humans are closer to chimpanzees than to gorillas or orangutans (**Figure 8**).

In this "DNA-DNA hybridization," the DNA of two species was cut into small chunks of 600–800 bp before mixing. Unfortunately, this technology was unable to prevent errors that were caused by the existence of paralogous sequences instead of orthologous sequences. The result was used for trending, similar to zoo-GISH, but it was not designed for accuracy. On the other hand, analyses that are focused on one or more genes that are present in the evolutionary history of only a few loci, lack a bridge to connect them. We are looking for a tool that is capable of not only whole genome and individual gene trending, but also larger block trending for

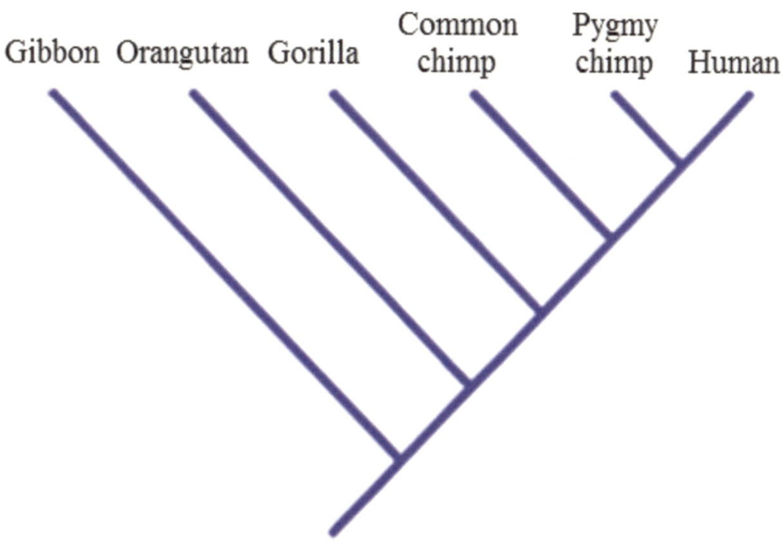

Figure 8. Phylogenetic relationship between Primates determined by DNA-DNA hybridization, modified from Ref. [9].

genomes, and even positioning. Therefore, the author chose to apply a mature technology from the study of human neoplasms called "metaphase comparative genomic hybridization (CGH)" to the study of phylogenetic history.

4. The history and prior applications of CGH

In 1992, Dan Pinkel's lab at UC San Francisco published an innovative technology named CGH [10]. In this method, tumor and normal cellular DNA probes were labeled with red and green fluorescence, respectively. They were then hybridized with normal cells in metaphase and competed with each other in incorporating with normal chromosomes. Yellow is observed when red and green fluorescence are mixed in equal amounts. A block with more tumor cell genome than the normal reference, i.e., with duplication, turns green, whereas deletion causes it to turn red. This innovative genome-wide technology not only allows positioning, but shows increase or decrease, making it a powerful tool in searching for tumor suppressing genes (which make the amount of tumor cells lower than those of normal reference) or oncogenes (which make the amount of tumor cells higher than those of normal reference), with a resolution of 5–10 Mbp. However, this technology is difficult to operate and requires specific photographic tools and image processing software to calculate the ratio of red and green fluorescence. Recently, gene chips have replaced this technology. Gene chips, formally known as array CGH (the original CGH was renamed as metaphase CGH), have designated probes that are fixed onto a chip [11]. The array CGH probes are derived from the known sequences of target organisms. Array CGH does not involve chromosomal preparation or microscope interpretation. Conversely, metaphase CGH is genome-wide and has chromosome-level resolution, and it is a useful tool when the full genome sequence is unknown. This technology can be applied in more than tumor research; it is also valuable for studying human genetic diseases that are related to repeated or deleted blocks, especially those that are caused by copy number variation [12]. The captured images and the last interpretation are presented in **Figure 9**, where (A) fluorescein (FITC) is used to provide green light; (B) rhodamine for red light; and (C) merged CGH results from one normal sample.

The fluorescence of the green-red ratio was analyzed with software.

We also applied this technology to report a rare case of missing human 13q31 without clinical symptoms [13]. In **Figure 10**, we can see that the human 13q31 block presents more red fluorescence in the block indicated by a straight red line (considered an increase when the green-red ratio is more than 1.2 and a decrease when the ratio is less than 0.8). The label n =18 indicates that the number of Chromosome 13 samples is 18. Therefore, 13q31 is possibly a large polymorphic block in the human genome and this discovery is important in clinical genetic consultations.

Based on the experience of metaphase CGH in human medicine, the author considered the feasibility of applying this technology in interspecies exploration to characterize the

http://dx.doi.org/10.5772/intechopen.68566

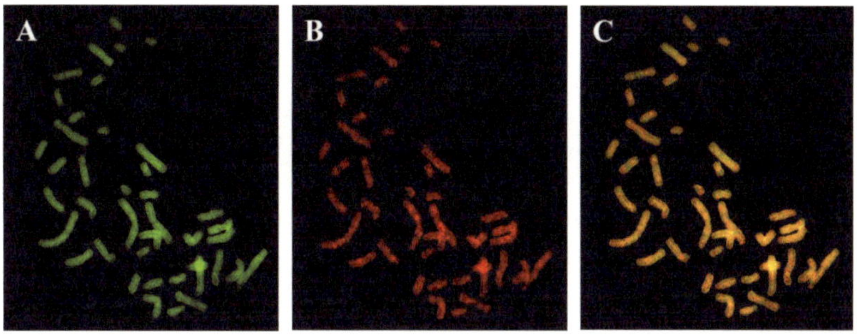

Figure 9. The result of metaphase CGH. (A) The signal of FITC-labeled probes. (B) The signal of rhodamine-labeled probes. (C) The merged CGH image of FITC and rhodamine.

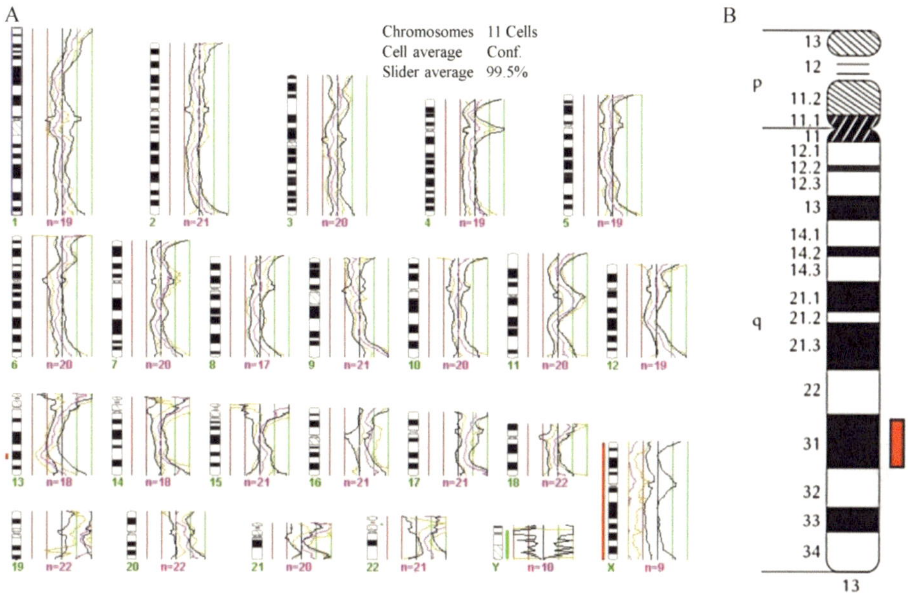

Figure 10. Metaphase CGH profiles of the 13q31 deletion case. (A) An interstitial deletion at band 13q31 was found (denoted as a red vertical bar beside chromosome 13). (B) An amplified ideogram of chromosome 13 with the deleted region marked by a red vertical bar on the right.

evolutionary relationships among extant eutherian mammalian taxonomic groups (orders/supraordinal clades). That is, to determine the sequence/genomic similarity of unknown-sequence species A and B with respect to species C, the DNA of species A and B would be labeled with molecules emitting different fluorescence dyes. The ratio of the labeled fluorescence intensities in each chromosome of species C should then reflect regions of sequence similarity to species A versus B. This is a brand-new application and the author named it "zoo-CGH" (**Figure 11**).

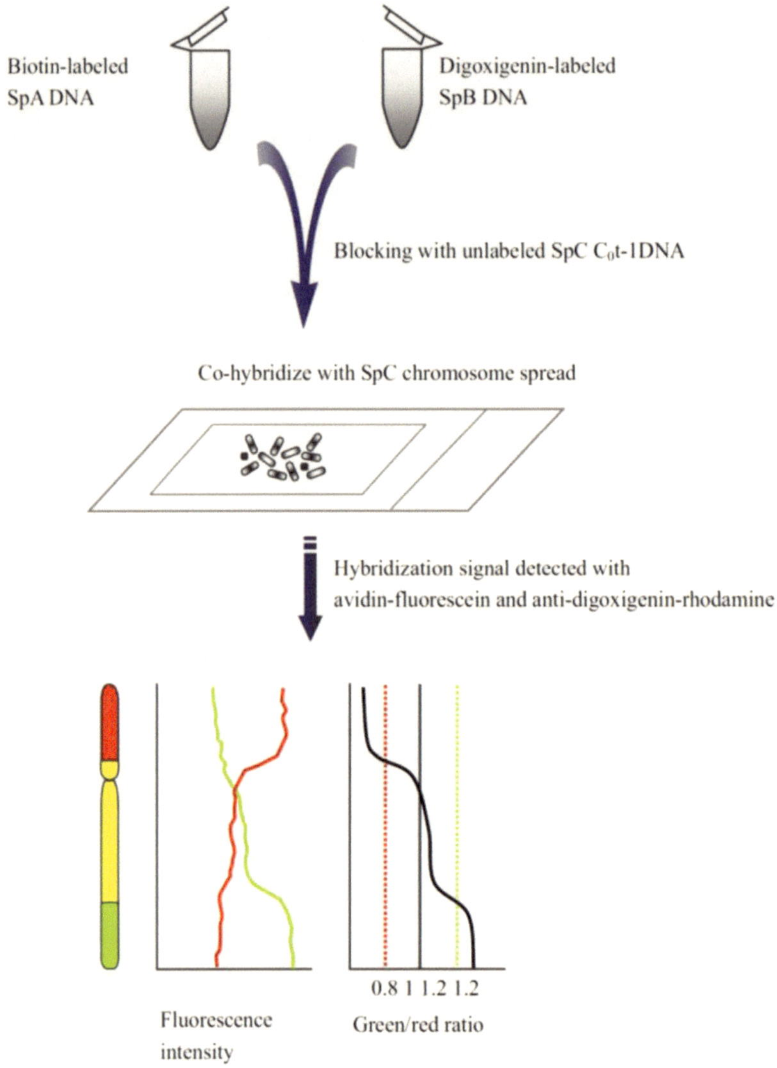

Figure 11. Schematic diagram of zoo-CGH. After calibration for genome size, equal amounts of genomic DNA from Species A (SpA) and Species B (SpB), labeled with a green and red fluorophore, respectively, were competitively hybridized to metaphase spreads of Species C (SpC).

5. Applying CGH in exploring the relationship between *Pholidota*, *Carnivora*, and *Xenarthra*

Myrmecophagy is a feeding behavior characterized by mainly or exclusively eating ants, termites, or both. This feeding specialization occurs in few eutherian mammals. Myrmecophagous species of Eutheria are in the orders Pholidota (e.g., pangolins, *Manis* spp, Manidae), Tubulidentata (e.g., aardvark, *Orycteropus afer*, Orycteropodidae) and Carnivora (e.g., aardwolf, *Proteles cristata*,

Hyaenidae), and superorder Xenarthra (e.g., anteaters, Myrmecophaga spp, Myrmecophagidae; armadillos, Dasypus spp, Dasypodidae) [14, 15]. These species share similar adaptations for this feeding specialization, including short teeth and jaws, a long sticky tongue, powerful forelimbs with strong claws, a rounded skull, and a low metabolic rate. In these species, the taxonomic status of Pholidota is a controversial issue. Morphological cladistics propose a close relationship between Pholidota and Xenarthra, whereas molecular evidence from mitochondrial and nuclear genes indicate that Pholidota is the sister taxa of Carnivora. However, it was recently noted that Pholidota lacks one of the lineage-specific karyotypic signatures of Carnivora. Zoo-CGH provided a genome-wide perspective on the relationship among Pholidota, Xenarthra, and Carnivora, even though the sequences of these animals are not fully determined. In the following example, DNA of the domestic dog (*Canis lupus familiaris*; Carnivora) and the two-toed sloth (*Choloepus didactylus*; Xenarthra) are labeled with different fluorophores and then hybridized with the metaphase chromosome spreads of Taiwanese pangolin (*Manis pentadactyla pentadactyla*; Pholidota).

5.1. Method and procedures

5.1.1. Determine nuclear genome size

The genome size of the two-toed sloth and domestic dog were determined to ensure that approximately equal numbers of nuclei (i.e., copy number of whole genomes in each species) are used in zoo-CGH analyses. The genome sizes were obtained after flow cytometry analysis of propidium iodide (IP)-stained nuclei from the target organisms.

5.1.2. Extract DNA from the two-toed sloth and domestic dog

Genomic DNA was isolated from leukocytes with a commercial kit (Gentra Puregene DNA Purification Kit, Qiagen, Hilden, German), used in accordance with the manufacturer's instructions.

5.1.3. Prepare the mitotic metaphase slides of Taiwanese pangolin

Fibroblast cell lines were established from lung tissues derived from Taiwanese pangolin, and metaphase cells were harvested following a 2-hour incubation with colcemid (at a concentration of 0.1 μg/ml).

5.1.4. Produce two-toed sloth and domestic dog DNA probes

The two-toed sloth and domestic dog DNA were labeled with biotin and digoxigenin (DIG) by nick translation, respectively.

5.1.5. Prepare pangolin C_0t-1 DNA

C_0t-1 DNA obtained its name from its isolation using a method called C_0t analysis (C_0 denotes "DNA concentration," whereas t denotes "time"). Repetitive nucleotide sequences, which constitute most of the C_0t-1 DNA, are abundantly distributed in most mammalian genomes. Blocking the repetitive sequences by C_0t-1 DNA can suppress nonspecific hybridization in FISH and CGH assays, and hence is a common step in such analyses. The genomic DNA of Taiwanese pangolin was sonicated to break the DNA into approximately 500-bp fragments, and the fragmented DNA was purified by ethanol precipitation. The purified DNA was dissolved to 500 ng/ml in TB buffer, denatured at 95°C for 10 minutes, and then chilled in ice for 10 minutes. A 1/10 volume of 12× SSC was then added to the fragmented DNA, which was reannealed at 60°C for 10 minutes. Then, S1-nuclease was used to digest the nonannealed DNA at 42°C for 1 hour. Thereafter, DNA was precipitated with ethanol and resuspended in TE buffer. Lastly, the acquired C_0t-1 DNA was quantified by spectrometry.

5.1.6. Perform zoo-CGH

Male Taiwanese pangolin chromosome spreads were prepared on a slide and denatured at 73°C for 5 minutes in 70% formamide and 2 × SSC, pH 7.0, followed by dehydration in a graded ethanol series. Next, equal genome copy numbers of biotin-labeled two-toed sloth DNA and DIG-labeled domestic dog DNA were coprecipitated with a 50-fold excess of Taiwanese pangolin C_0t-1 DNA, then redissolved in 10 μl of hybridization buffer (50% formamide, 10% dextran sulfate, and 2 × SSC), acting as the hybridization probe. Before hybridization, the probe was denatured at 80°C for 7 minutes, and then incubated at 37°C for 1 hour for preannealing of the repetitive DNA. The denatured probe was applied to the slide with the denatured and dehydrated metaphase spreads, covered with a cover slip, sealed, and incubated at 37°C for 72 hours. After hybridization, the slide was washed three times with 50% formamide and 2% SSC at 40°C for 5 minutes, and then washed twice with 2% SSC at 40°C for 5 minutes. The slide was kept undisturbed with 0.1% Tween 20 in 4 × SSC for 5 minutes, and the hybridization signal was detected with fluorescein-conjugated avidin (green fluorescence; for biotin-labeled probe) and rhodamine-conjugated ant-DIG antibody (red fluorescence; for DIG-labeled probe). Pangolin chromosomes were counterstained with 4′, 6-diamidino-2-phenylindole (DAPI) and fluorescence signals were visualized under a Leica DMLB microscope equipped with a cooled CCD camera. The profile of the fluorescein versus rhodamine fluorescence intensity ratio (F/R ratio) was estimated with CGHView image analysis software.

5.1.7. Analyze image

By comparing the fluorescence ratio on the longitudinal axis of pangolin metaphase chromosome, we estimated differences in the inter-species gene copy number and DNA sequence similarity. The means of the F/R ratios obtained from the heterologous hybridization, which represents DNA from different species labeled with different fluorophores that are competitively bound to probes obtained from a third species, were calculated for each pangolin autosome. Pangolin chromosomal segments with F/R ratios of < 0.8 (red fluorescence is more intense) and > 1.2 (green fluorescence is more intense) were considered to have significantly different hybridization strengths. When the F/R ratios were between 0.8 and 1.2 (showing yellow fluorescence), the DNA sequence difference or copy number of each pair was roughly equivalent. Means of the ratios were also calculated using a dye-swap design.

5.2. Result

In **Figure 12**, we can see red, green or yellow blocks on different parts of the chromosome. The overall homology between the pangolin and dog genomes was higher than that between the pangolin and sloth genomes. Analysis of pangolin chromosomes 14 and 15, which were the largest and most easily identifiable, showed that red fluorescence is dominant in euchromatin, i.e., more similar to the domestic dog (**Figure 12E**). When dye swapping was conducted, i.e., green fluorescence for the domestic dog and red fluorescence for the two-toed sloth, consistent results were obtained (**Figure 12F**).

Figure 12 shows zoo-CGH for the domestic dog, two-toed sloth, and Taiwanese pangolin. In panel (A) genomic DNA from dog (labeled with DIG conjugated to the red fluorophore, rhodamine) and sloth (labeled with biotin conjugated to the green fluorophore, fluorescein) were mixed in equal quantities and competitively hybridized to metaphase spreads from the pangolin lymphocytes. In panel (B) individual chromosome analysis of the fluorescent ratio in (A) was presented where blue lines denote the ratio of F/R signal at each position of the pangolin chromosomes. Numbers in brackets represent the number of chromosomes analyzed. When the vertical bar between each chromosome and its ideogram appears red or green, the F/R ratio was <0.8 or >1.2, respectively. Overall, all chromosomes (except Y) appeared red. Panels (C) and (D) represent dye swap of (A) and (B), respectively. All chromosomes (except Y) appeared green.

From the results above, we found that all somatic chromosomes of *Manis pentadactyla* are more similar to the domestic dog (Carnivora) than the two-toed sloth (Xenarthra), providing evidence that *Pholidota* is more related to Carnivora than Xenarthra. For the Y chromosomes, which show the opposite results, we must eliminate the possibility of deletion of domestic dog's Y chromosome. We further analyzed the karyotype of this individual, but did not find such deletion. Therefore, it is possible that Y chromosome of *Manis pentadactyla* has a different evolutionary history than the somatic chromosomes [16]. The differences in the Y chromosome results can also be attributed to the size difference between the Y chromosomes of domestic dog and two-toed sloth. The large genomic blocks of somatic chromosomes lack structural rearrangements during evolution, making "richness" prevail in signal expression instead of "similarity," which is more desired. We performed molecular evolution analysis with the *Sry* gene, which is located on Y chromosome, and the results were combined with those from zoo-CGH; that is, two markers of different evolutionary history were used to answer the question. There is no doubt in the answer: in terms of extant mammal taxonomy, Pholidota has a closer relationship with Carnivora than Xenarthra. The new methods we developed can be used as a powerful tool for clarifying the phylogenetic relationships of orders under the Mammalia class, and they help answer some long-disputed taxonomical questions. For example, to which greater taxonomical category should Chiroptera belong: Laurasiatheria or Euarchontoglires? Zoo-CGH not only reveals the similarity trend of the whole genome but also individual gene blocks, making it the CGH technology with the highest resolution before the complete sequencing of each species; when it is combined with cross-species whole chromosome painting FISH (zoo-FISH), a new era of comparative genomics begins [17].

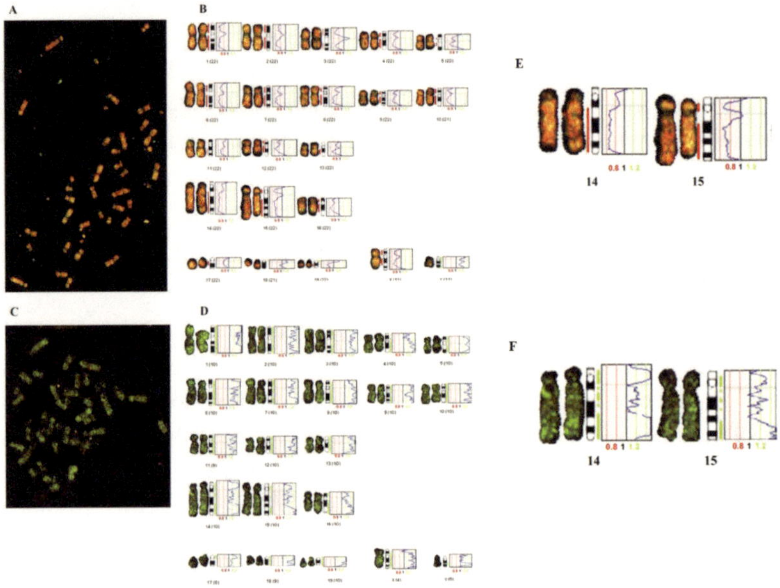

Figure 12. Cross-species CGH for the domestic dog (*Canis lupus*), two-toed sloth (*Chloepus didactylus*), and Taiwanese pangolin (*Manis pentadactyla pentadactyla*). (A) The competitively hybridization results of dog (rhodamine) and sloth (FITC) to metaphase spreads from pangolin lymphocytes. (B) Individual chromosome analysis of the fluorescent ratio in (A). (C) and (D) dye swap of (A) and (B), respectively. (E) and (F) Enlarge pangolin chromosomes 14 and 15 of (B) and (D), respectively.

6. Discussion

In early times, comparative genomics study between closely related species can only be done by comparing the karyotypes of the species and the techniques used are primitive, including Giemsa stain only, the G-banding techniques, and thus only the diploid number (2N), the functional number (FN, indicating the numbers of the chromosomal arms), as well as the classification of the chromosomes into metacentric, submetacentric, acrocentric, and telocentric according to the arm ratios can be provided. In addition, the special stains, such as the C-banding and Ag-nucleolus organizer region (NOR) staining, can be used to elucidate the constitutive heterochromatin (by C-banding), and the sites of secondary constriction and the active-transcribing ribosomal DNA genes (by Ag-NOR staining), can help to find the more trivial differences between species which may carry evolutionary significance [18, 19]. However, the advent of fluorescence *in situ* hybridization (FISH) technology greatly expanded the role of cytogenetics in studying the karyotypic evolution, not only in mammals but also in plants [5, 7, 20]. The authors therefore propose here a complete cytogenetic study in the light of karyotypic evolution that should include the conventional karyotyping, the special stains, as well as the fluorescence *in situ* hybridization (FISH)-based technologies such as genomic *in situ* hybridization (which is specific to plants), the chromosomal painting to study the movement and shuffling of the large genomic blocks in the Mb-level (in mammals), the telomere (TTAGGG)*n* FISH to demarcate the

http://dx.doi.org/10.5772/intechopen.68566

chromosomal ends or to demonstrate the insertional translocation between species (in all vertebrates), mapping the locations of the gene of special interest with the FISH probe made by the gene segment cloned (in both animals and plants), and the innovative zoo-CGH we described in the previous section (in mammals), as our previous studies recently demonstrated [17–19].

7. Conclusion

Despite molecular evolution being made nowadays, by studying the homologous DNA sequences and using different evolutionary analytical models to reconstruct the phylogeny, which is the mainstream of comparative genomics [1–4], especially when sequencing the whole genome of each species has become more feasible through the powerful next generation sequencing (NGS) technology [21], cytogenetics remains an indispensible tool in studying the karyotypic evolution, which is one of the major mechanisms and thus is equally important as the molecular evolution to the processes involved in the speciation and subspecies differentiation. Conventional karyotyping, special stains to delineate the locations of heterochromatin, sites of active-transcribing ribosomal DNA genes, as well as molecular cytogenetics (namely, the fluorescence *in situ* hybridization (FISH)-based methodologies) can still provide insightful clues to solve the deficiencies that molecular evolution-based analyses cannot easily answer because in addition to point mutations and small insertion/deletions (indels), the movement of large genomic segments in the size of Mb-level, which is very difficult to analyze if by molecular methods, is also important in the evolution of the genetic complements of species deriving from a common ancestor in a specific lineage. The authors therefore propose a more balanced approach to study phylogenetics that is mandatory when considering using cytogenetics or molecular analyses as the major research tool. Evolutionary genetics will not be complete if the valuable insights obtained through cytogenetics are ignored or omitted in this NGS-predominant molecular era.

Author details

Ming Chen[1,2,3,4]*, Wen-Hsiang Lin[1,2], Dong-Jay Lee[1,2], Shun-Ping Chang[1,2], Tze-Ho Chen[4] and Gwo-Chin Ma[1,2]

*Address all correspondence to: mchen_cch@yahoo.com

1 Department of Genomic Medicine, and Core Lab for System Biology, Changhua Christian Hospital, Changhua, Taiwan

2 Department of Genomic Science and Technology, Changhua Christian Hospital, Changhua, Taiwan

3 Department of Obstetrics and Gynecology, College of Medicine, National Taiwan University, Taipei, Taiwan

4 Department of Life Science, Tunghai University, Taichung, Taiwan

References

[1] Springer MS, Murphy WJ, Eizirik E, O'Brien SJ. Placental mammal diversification and the Cretaceous-Tertiary boundary. Proceedings of the National Academy of Sciences of the United States of America. 2003;**100**:1056-1061. DOI: 10.1073/pnas.0334222100

[2] Murphy WJ, Eizirik E, Johnson WE, Zhang YP, Ryder OA, O'Brien SJ. Molecular phylogenetics and the origins of the placental mammals. Nature. 2001;**409**:614-618. DOI: 10.1038/35054550

[3] Murphy WJ, Larkin DM, Wind AE, Bourque G, Tesler G, Auvil L, Beever JE, Chowdhary Bp, Galibert F, Gatzke L, Hitte C, Meyers SN, Milan D, Ostrnder EA, Pape G, Parker HG, Raudsepp T, Rogatcheva MB, Schook LB, Skow LC, Welge M, Womack JE, O'Brien SJ, Pevzner PA, Lewin HA. Dynamics of mammalian chromosome evolution inferred from multispecies comparative maps. Science. 2005;**309**:613-617. DOI: 10.1126/science.1111387

[4] Murphy WJ, Stanyon R, O'Brien SJ. Evolution of mammalian genome organization inferred from comparative gene mapping. Genome Biology. 2001b;**2**(6):reviews0005.1-reviews0005.8. DOI: 10.1186/gb-2001-2-6-reviews0005

[5] Ferguson-Smith MA, Yang F, RensW, O'Brien PC. The impact of chromosome sorting and painting on the comparative analysis of primate genomes. Cytogenetic and Genome Research. 2005;**108**(1-3):112-121. DOI: 10.1159/000080809

[6] Burt DW, Bruley C, Dunn IC, Jones CT, Ramage A, Law AS, Morrice DR, Paton IR, Smith J, Windsor D, Sazanov A, Fries R, Waddington D. The dynamics of chromosome evolution in birds and mammals. Nature. 1999;**402**:411-413. DOI: 10.1038/46555

[7] Svartman M, Stone G, Stanyon R. The ancestral eutherian karyotype is present in Xenarthra. PLoS Genetics. 2006;**2**(7):e109. DOI: 10.1371/journal.pgen.0020109

[8] Amrin-Madsen H, Koepfli KP, Wayne RK, Springer MS. A new phylogenetic marker, Apolipoprotein B, provides compelling evidence for eutherian relationships. Molecular Phylogenetics and Evolution. 2003;**28**(2):225-240. DOI: 10.1016/S1055-7903(03)00118-0

[9] Sibley CG, Ahlquist JE. The phylogeny of the hominoid primates, as indicated by DNA-DNA hybridization. Journal of Molecular Evolution. 1984;**20**(1):2-15. DOI: 10.1007/BF02101980

[10] Kallioniemi A, Kallioniemi OP, Sudar D, Rutovitz D, Gray JW, Waldman F, Pinkel D. Comparative genomic hybridization for molecular cytogenetic analysis of solid tumors. Science. 1992;**258**(5083):818-821. DOI: 10.1126/science.1359641

[11] Kallioniemi A. CGH microarrays and cancer. Current Opinion in Biotechnology. 2008;**19**(1):36-40. DOI: 10.1016/j.copbio.2007.11.004

[12] Lee C, Iafrate AJ, Brothman AR. Copy number variations and clinical cytogenetic diagnosis of constitutional disorders. Nature Genetics. 2007;**39**(7 Suppl):S48-S54. DOI: 10.1038/ng2092

[13] Ke YY, Lee DJ, Ma GC, Lee MH, Wang BT, Chen M. Interstitial deletion 13q31 associated with normal phenotype: cytogenetic study of a family with concomitant segregation of reciprocal translocation and interstitial deletion. Journal of the Formosan Medical Association. 2007;**106**(7):582-588 DOI: 10.1016/S0929-6646(07)60010-2

[14] McNab BK. Physiological convergence amongst ant-eating and termite-eating mammals. Journal of Zoology. 1984;**203**:485-510. DOI: 10.1111/j.1469-7998.1984.tb02345.x

[15] Redford KH. Ant and termites as food: Patterns of mammalian myrmecophagy. In: Genoways HH, editor. Current Mammalogy. New York: Springer; 1987. pp. 349-399. DOI: 10.1007/978-1-4757-9909-5_9

[16] Yu HT, Ma GC, Lee DJ, Chin SC, Tsao HS, Wu SH, Shih SY, Chen M. Molecular delineation of the Y-borne Sry gene in the Formosan pangolin (*Manis pentadactyla pentadactyla*) and its phylogenetic implications for Pholidota in extant mammals. Theriogenology. 2011;**75**(1):55-64. DOI: 10.1016/j.theriogenology.2010.07.010

[17] Yu HT, Ma GC, Lee DJ, Chin SC, Chen TL, Tsao HS, Lin WH, Wu SH, Lin CC, Chen M. Use of a cytogenetic whole-genome comparison to resolve phylogenetic relationships among three species: Implications for mammalian systematics and conservation biology. Theriogenology. 2012;**77**(8):1615-1623. DOI: 10.1016/j.theriogenology.2011.12.006

[18] Wu SH, Chen M, Chin SC, Lee DJ, Wen PY, Chen LW, Wang BT, Yu HT. Cytogenetic analysis of the Formosan pangolin *Manis pentadactyla pentadactyla* (Mammalia: Pholidota). Zoological Studies. 2007;**46**:389-396

[19] Lin LK, Ma GC, Chen TH, Lin WH, Lee DJ, Wen PY, Wu SH, Chen M. Genomic analyses of the Formosan harvest mouse (Micromys minutus) and comparisons to the brown Norway rat (Rattus norvegicus) and the house mouse (Mus musculus). Zoology (Jena). 2013;**116**(5):307-315. DOI: 10. 1016/j.zool.2013.07.001

[20] Silva GS, Souza MM. Genomic in situ hybridization in plants. Genetics and Molecular Research 2013;**12**(3):2953-2965. DOI: 10.4238/2013.August.12.11

[21] Pennisi E. Sequencing all life captivates biologists. Science. 2017;**355**(6328):894-895. DOI: 10.1126/Science.355.6328.894

Chapter 5

Phylogenetic and Functional Diversity of Faecal Microbiome of Pack Animals

Suchitra Sena Dande, Niteen V. Patil and Chaitanya G. Joshi

Additional information is available at the end of the chapter

http://dx.doi.org/10.5772/intechopen.69252

Abstract

The present chapter describes the microbial diversity of faecal microbiomes of pack animals. The sequencing data generated through ion semiconductor sequencing technology were analysed using EBI metagenomics and MG-RAST server tools. Bacteria were the major domain in all the pack animals. At the phylogenetic level, Firmicutes was the major phylum. Clostridiales was the major order. *Ruminococcus flavefaciens* was the major species in camel, whereas the top-most species existing in Equidae family was *Streptococcus equinus*. Among the 28 major functional categories, protein metabolism functionality was dominant in pack animals. The genes associated with protein processing and modification as well as for protein folding are higher in mules and in camel they are lowest. Central carbohydrate metabolism was the major functional group under carbohydrate metabolism in pack animals. Variation in the amino acids and its derivatives was seen in pack animals. Genes associated with proline and 4-hydroxy prolines were present in Equidae family only. Clustering using ward with Bray-Curtis distance matrix for the functional categories showed that donkey and mule are most closely related and clustered with the horse metagenome.

Keywords: Camelidae, Equidae, faecal microbiome, taxonomic, functionality

1. Introduction

The pack animals, namely camel, horse, mule and donkey are traditionally regarded as animals for transportation/draught. Among pack animals, dromedary camel is a pseudo-ruminant and a foregut fermenter, while equidae members are non-ruminant hindgut fermenters. Anaerobic habitats have existed continuously throughout the history of the earth, the gastrointestinal tract being a contemporary microniche [1]. The microbial community inhabiting the gastrointestinal tract is represented by all major domains of microbes, including Bacteria, Archaea and Eucarya [2] as well as viruses (bacteriophage), and characterized by its high population density, wide diversity and complexity of interactions which play a vital role in the normal nutritional, physiological, immunological and protective functions of the host animal.

Literature shows [3–6] that 1–5% of the microbial diversity can be known through cultivation techniques. Over a period of time, advances from a culture-dependent to culture-independent technologies have revolutionized understanding the microbial ecology. Metagenomics or culture-independent genomic analysis helps to understand the biology of uncultured bacteria, archaea and viruses which can unveil the genetic diversity, population structure and ecology in particular environmental niche [7]. As sequencing costs continue to diminish, the breadth of metagenomic research increases. The sequencing technology and bioinformatics have enabled the molecular characterization of gastrointestinal microbial populations in livestock. Metagenomics helps in visualizing the complex microbial communities which have impact on the health of animals and human and global biogeochemical cycles [8–10]. Next-generation sequencing technologies were being used to characterize the microbial diversity and functional capacity of a range of microbial communities in the gastrointestinal tracts of several animal species [11–18]. Understanding the genetic composition of faecal microbial communities does have implications on food and water safety and animal faeces can also harbour human pathogens. The personal genome machine (PGM) platforms provide a low-cost, scalable and high-throughput solution for studying the microbial community structure and function analyses [19].

2. Methodology

Upon the ethical committee approval, faecal samples from pack animals (camel, horse, mule and donkey) were collected from rectum and immediately placedon ice and stored at -80°C till further DNA extraction; 250 mg of faecal material was subjected for lysis and DNA was extracted by the using QIAmp DNA stool mini kit (Qiagen, USA). The DNA purity and concentration was analysed by spectrophotometric quantification and gel electrophoresis. Enzymatic fragmentation was done to yield fragments of 280–300 bp size. Later library construction followed by emulsion polymerase chain reaction (ePCR) was done. The recovered ePCR product was loaded onto Ion torrent PGM 316 chip for sequencing as per manufacturer's instructions on Ion Torrent PGM. Generated data were uploaded on MG-RAST (the Metagenomics RAST) server. MG-RAST server [20] is an automated platform for the analysis of microbial metagenomes to get the quantitative insights of the microbial populations. Metagenomic comparisons were made with the yet-to-publicize metagenomic data sets of camel (4513857.3), horse (4514961.3), mule (4514940.3) and donkey (4514220.3) on MG-RAST Server. The Post QC data were also submitted to EBI metagenomics [21] in the projects camel (ERS631575), horse (ERS631759), mule (ERS631825) and donkey (ERS631580) for comparing the microbial diversity which are yet to be publicized. The maximum e-value of 1e-5, minimum per cent identity of 80 and minimum alignment length of 50 bp for 16SrRNA taxonomy and 30 bp for functionalities were applied as the parameter settings in the analysis. Clustering was performed using Ward's minimum variance with Bray-Curtis distance matrix for normalized values on MG-RAST analysis was done.

3. Faecal microbial diversity

3.1. Diversity of the camel faecal metagenome sequences

The summary of the sequencing datasets uploaded on MG-RAST is shown in **Table 1**.

3.2. Taxonomic classification

The phylogenetic data revealed bacteria as the major domain in all pack animals. Firmicutes was the major phylum. A total of 22–31% of reads were unassigned bacterial phylum. In camels, higher Firmicutes to Bacteroides ratio of 3.8 was observed, whereas in horse, mule and donkey the ratio was 1.5, 1.6 and 1.7, respectively. The difference in the microbial diversity at the phylum level may be due to the variations in digestive physiology of camels and equines. **Figure 1** represents the per cent abundance of operational taxonomic units (OTUs) at phylum level. Fusobacteria and Fibrobacteres phyla were exclusively observed in donkey, whereas WPS-2, Actinobacteria, and Elusimicrobia were found exclusively in mule, camel and horse, respectively. In mules, >10% of the reads were assigned to Verrucomicrobia phylum. In human beings, the *Firmicutes/Bacteroidetes* ratio undergoes an increase from birth to adulthood and is further altered with advanced age [22]. *Verrucomicrobia* is a universally distributed phylum and first observed in freshwater [23]; this phylum has already been discovered in termite gut, human intestines and sea cucumbers as well as in very extreme environments [24]. All the pack animals showed this phylum with high abundance in mules. Comparative analyses of 16S rRNA gene sequences prepared from the foregut contents of 12 adult feral camels in Australia fed on native vegetation also observed that the majority of bacteria were affiliated to phylum Firmicutes. The remaining phyla were represented by Actinobacteria, Chloroflexi, Cynophyta, Lentisphaerae, Planctomycetes, Proteobacteria and Sphirochaetes [25]. The taxonomic analysis of metagenomic reads indicated Bacteroidetes (55.5%), Firmicutes (22.7%) and

Metagenome id		Camel	Horse	Mule	Donkey
Post QC data	bp count (bp)	55,194,766	43,405,015	81,917,010	41,499,354
	Sequence count ORF's	385,464	321,769	561,418	275,682
	Mean sequence length (bp)	143 ± 63	134 ± 61	145 ± 63	150 ± 65
	Mean GC per cent (%)	46 ± 10	46 ± 9	47 ± 10	47 ± 9
Predicted	Protein features	306,905	256,458	461,826	233,866
	rRNA features	73,473	55,421	95,936	43,902
Identified	Protein features	132,735	104,681	177,488	96,095
	rRNA features	843	523	910	854
	Functional categories	80,877	64,961	109,704	58,412

Table 1. Summary of analysed data of faecal metagaenomes of pack animals.

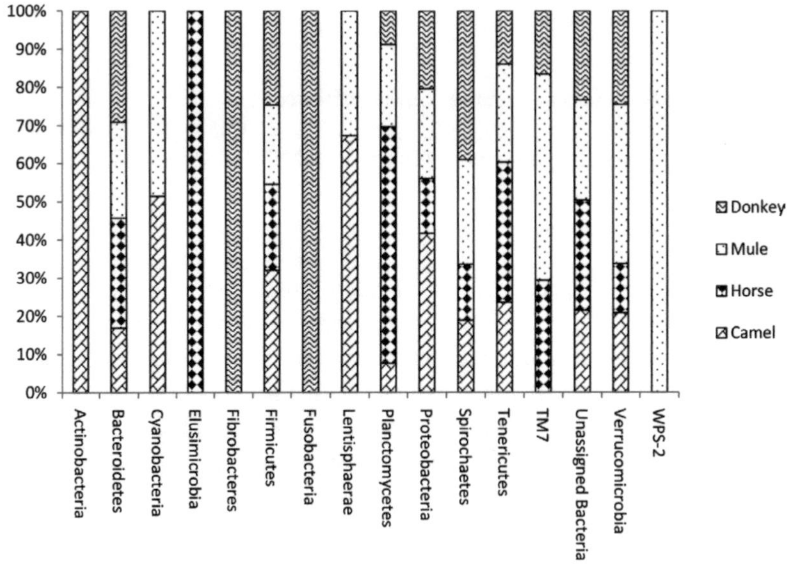

Figure 1. Per cent abundant OTUs of different phyla in pack animals.

Proteobacteria (9.2%) phyla as predominant camel rumen taxa and *Bacteroides* species dominated the camel rumen metagenome [26]. But in the faecal metagenome, Firmicutes was the major phylum in camel. The alteration in the part of the digestive tract does have influence on its microbial diversity.

The phylogenetic resolution at order, genus and species was assigned a maximum e-value of 1×10^{-5}, a minimum identity of 80% and a minimum alignment length of 50 bp using M5RNA data base within MG-RAST. Microbial diversity at the order level revealed more microbes in Clostridiales (>50%) followed by Bacteroidales (>10%) in camel. In horses, Clostridiales (38.2%) followed by Lactobacillales (22.9%) and Bacteroidales (11.4%) were the predominant orders. In mules and donkeys, Clostridiales (39.9 and 43.2%) followed by Bacteroidales (16.2 and 17.5%) and Lactobacillales (8.5 and 14.5%) were the predominant orders. At the genus level, Clostridium was the major organism in mule and camel, while Streptococcus was most abundant in horse and donkey. The top-most genera (>1%) were shown in **Figure 2a–d**. In camels, *Ruminococcus flavefaciens* is the most abundant species and in all equidae members *Streptococcus equinus* is the major organism at species level.

3.3. Predicted gene functions

The data were analysed using SEED subsystem within MG-RAST. An overview of the predicted functions of genes sequenced from pack animals was presented in **Table 2**. Twenty-eight functional categories were assigned with maximum per cent of genes assigned for protein metabolism in all pack animals (>10%). The study on camel rumen functional analysis revealed that clustering-based subsystem and carbohydrate metabolism were the most abundant SEED subsystem representing 17 and 13% of camel metagenome, respectively [26].

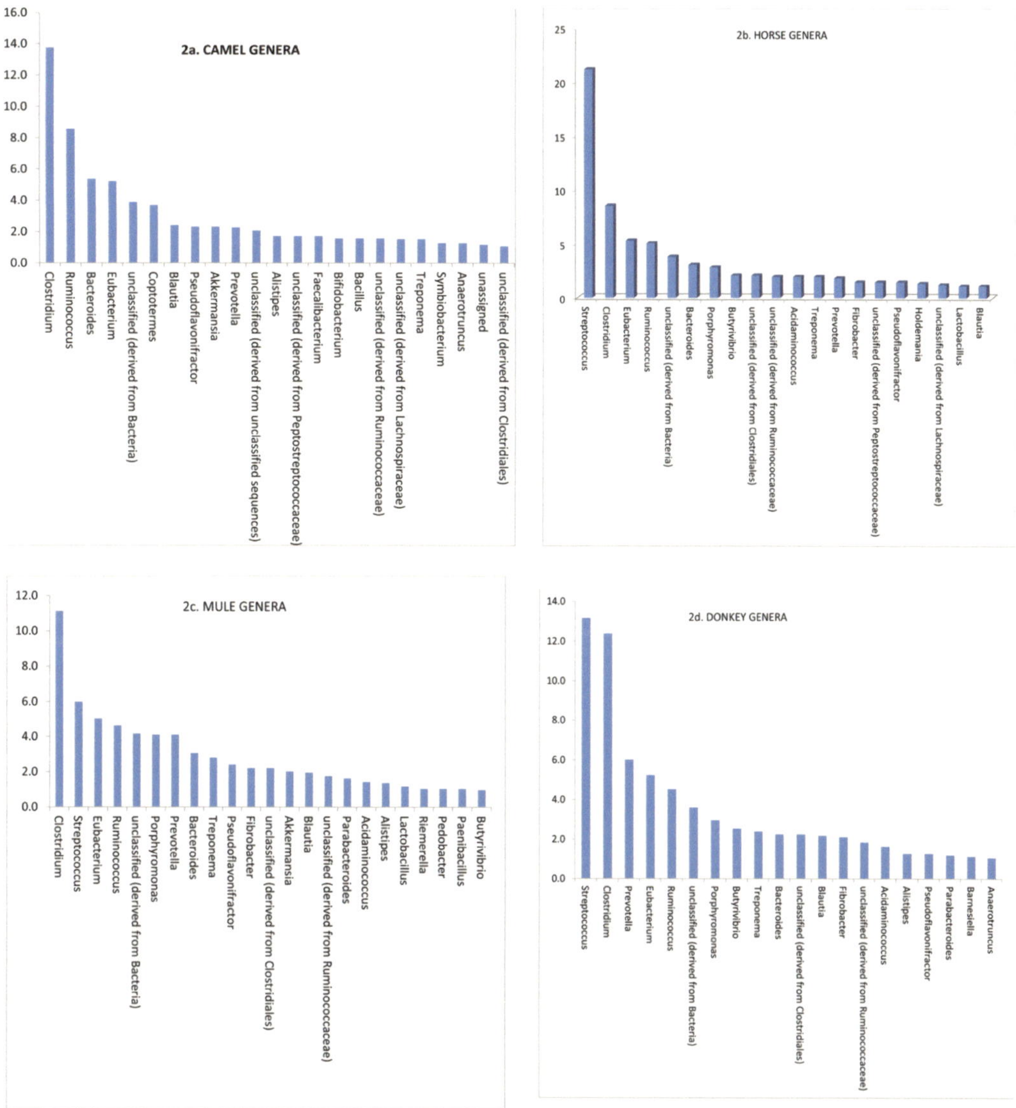

Figure 2. (a–d) Per cent abundance of different genera in pack animals (>1%). The data were compared to M5RNA using a maximum e-value of 1e–5, a minimum identity of 80% and a minimum alignment length of 50 measured in bp for RNA databases.

3.3.1. Protein metabolism

In protein metabolism, the sub-category of genes associated with protein biosynthesis showed high abundance in all pack animals (**Figure 3**). Among the genes associated for protein metabolism, the genes of protein degradation were highest in horses (12.9%) and lowest in mules (1.2%). In mule, a high percentage of genes for protein processing and modification as well as for protein folding were observed and in camel they were lowest.

Functional categories	Camel	Horse	Mule	Donkey
Amino acids and derivatives	7.9	4.7	3.9	4.3
Carbohydrates	8.7	8.8	10.6	8.9
Cell division and cell cycle	1.3	0.7	1.2	0.9
Cell wall and capsule	2.3	1.8	3.0	2.6
Clustering-based subsystems	7.4	8.7	7.2	6.4
Cofactors, vitamins, prosthetic groups, pigments	3.0	3.8	3.0	2.3
DNA metabolism	1.6	2.6	2.7	2.0
Dormancy and sporulation	0.1	0.1	0.1	0.1
Fatty acids, lipids, and isoprenoids	1.8	1.7	2.4	1.8
Iron acquisition and metabolism	0.2	0.2	0.2	0.1
Membrane transport	3.0	5.7	2.8	2.5
Metabolism of aromatic compounds	2.3	2.9	1.1	1.9
Miscellaneous	7.0	7.9	4.7	7.2
Motility and chemotaxis	1.6	0.9	2.3	1.5
Nitrogen metabolism	1.2	1.8	1.9	1.7
Nucleosides and nucleotides	3.5	3.7	3.4	3.5
Phages, prophages, transposable elements, plasmids	4.3	4.5	3.5	4.6
Phosphorus metabolism	0.1	0.4	0.2	0.9
Photosynthesis	0.5	0.5	0.7	0.5
Potassium metabolism	0.5	0.1	0.3	0.0
Protein metabolism	11.1	11.0	13.6	14.7
RNA metabolism	10.4	9.6	9.3	10.7
Regulation and cell signalling	2.7	3.3	2.5	3.5
Respiration	7.1	6.2	10.0	7.7
Secondary metabolism	2.4	1.5	0.9	0.6
Stress response	3.7	3.8	4.5	5.2
Sulphur metabolism	2.7	0.9	1.5	1.0
Virulence, disease and defence	1.7	2.3	2.6	3.0

Table 2. Per cent abundance of different functional categories in pack animals.

3.3.2. Carbohydrates

Central carbohydrate metabolism was the major functional group under carbohydrate metabolism in pack animals (**Figure 4**). The second richest functional group in carbohydrate metabolism was genes associated with carbon dioxide fixation in camel and mule and one-carbon metabolism in horse and donkey. Genes associated with one-carbon metabolism and fermentation were higher among all equidae members compared to camels. Glycoside hydrolases were seen exclusively in horses. Polysaccharide-associated genes were not seen in donkeys.

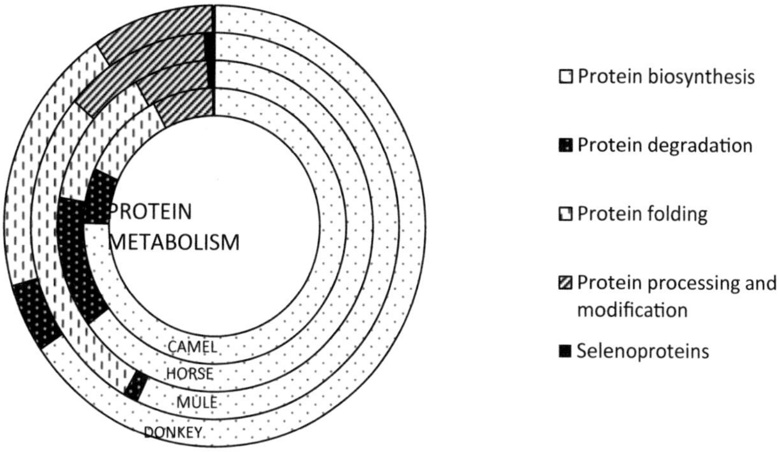

Figure 3. Per cent abundance of sub-categories in protein metabolism for pack animals. The data were compared to SEED subsystems using a maximum e-value of 1e–5, a minimum identity of 80% and a minimum alignment length of 30 measured in aa for protein.

3.3.3. *Amino acids and derivatives*

Amino acids and derivatives form one of the abundant functional categories in camels (7.9%) (**Figure 5**). The genes associated with aromatic amino acids and derivatives were higher in camels. Arginine, urea cycle and polyamines genes were higher in horse compared to others. In mule, genes associated for aromatic amino acids and derivatives as well as branched chain amino acids were higher compared to other sub-category genes. In donkeys, branched chain

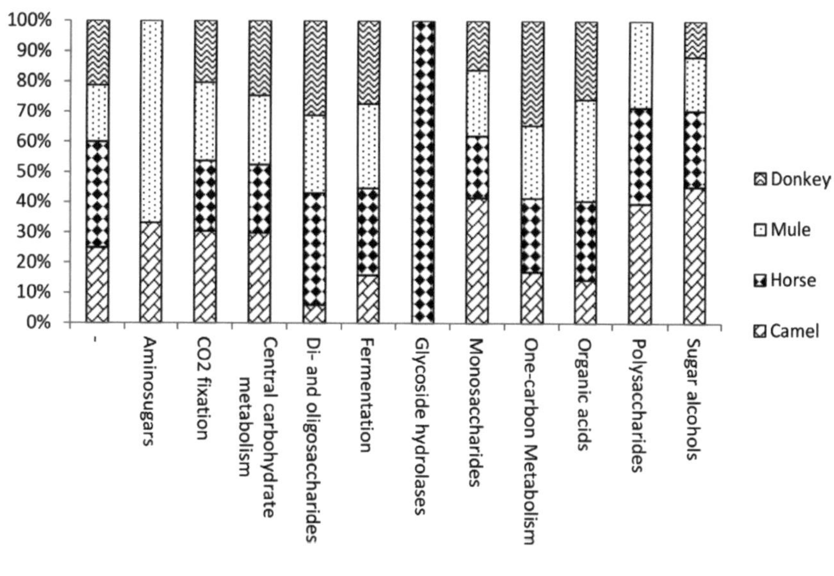

Figure 4. Per cent abundance of sub-categories in central carbohydrate metabolism for pack animals. The data were compared to SEED subsystems using a maximum e-value of 1e–5, a minimum identity of 80% and a minimum alignment length of 30 measured in aa for protein.

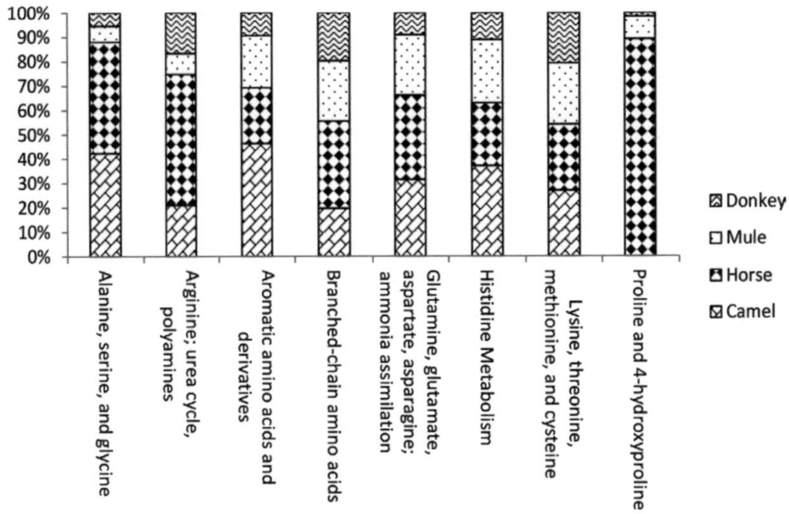

Figure 5. Per cent abundance of sub-categories in amino acids and derivatives for pack animals. The data were compared to SEED subsystems using a maximum e-value of 1e–5, a minimum identity of 80% and a minimum alignment length of 30 measured in aa for protein.

amino acids were higher. In camels, genes associated for proline and 4-hydroxyl proline metabolism were absent, lowest in mules and higher in horses.

3.3.4. *Virulence, disease and defence genes*

A suite of genes associated with resistance to antibiotic and toxic compounds (RATC) was highest in pack animals (**Figure 6**). The genes assigned for the virulence and antibiotic resistance

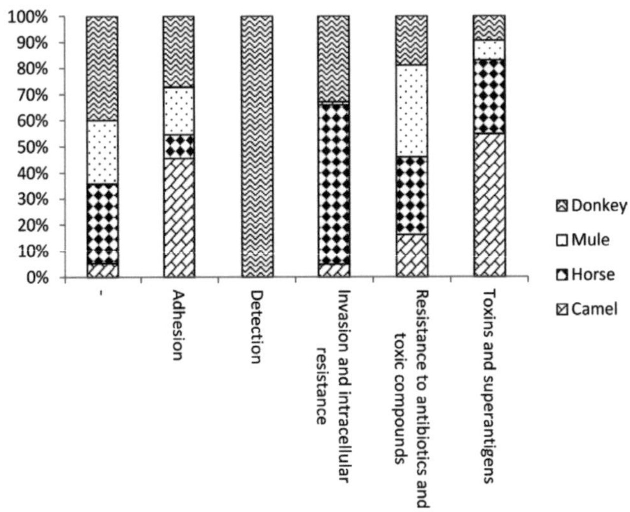

Figure 6. Per cent abundance of sub-categories in virulence, disease and defence for pack animals. The data were compared to SEED subsystems using a maximum e-value of 1e–5, a minimum identity of 80% and a minimum alignment length of 30 measured in aa for protein.

http://dx.doi.org/10.5772/intechopen.69252

revealed abundant FemC, factor associated with methicillin resistance in all pack animals. The sub-category of detection genes was seen only in donkeys.

3.4. Comparison of microbial diversity at taxonomic and functional levels in pack animals

Comparative taxonomic and functional similarity of the pack animal faecal metagenomes was compared for generating heat maps. Hierarchical clustering of taxonomic profiles of pack animals derived from faecal metagenomes revealed that horse and donkey are closely similar (**Figures 7**). Functional similarity of samples investigated in the present study revealed that donkey and mule are closely related (**Figures 8**). The comparative metagenomic approach used in this study identified unique and/or over-abundant taxonomic and functional elements within metagenome projects.

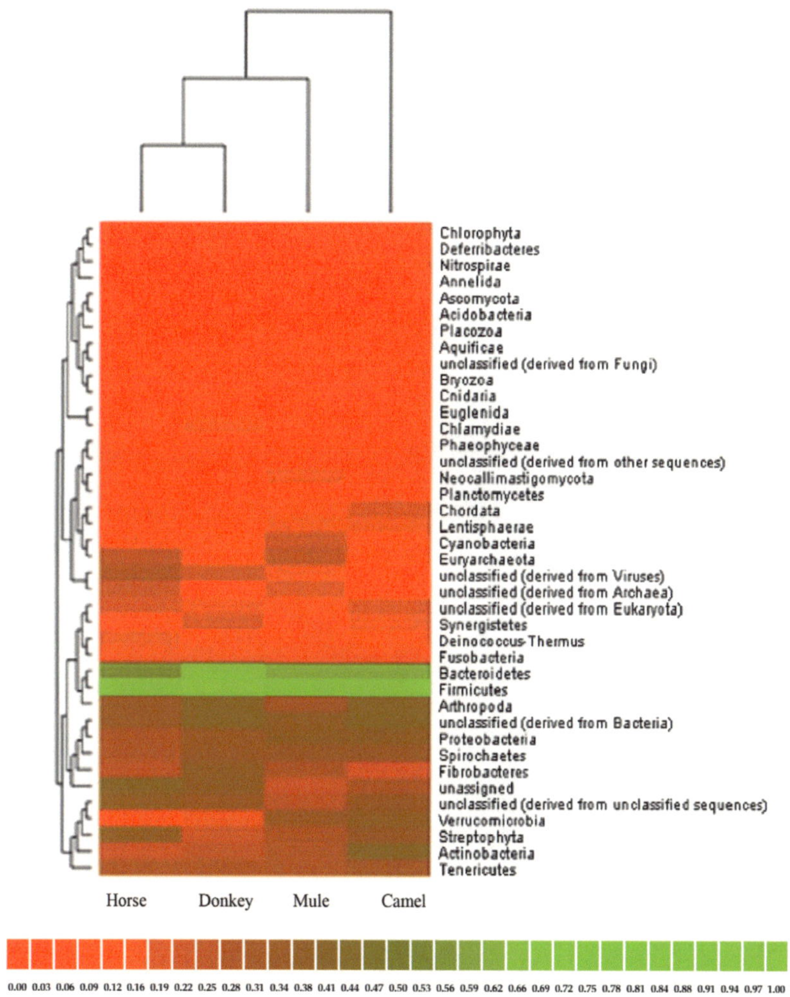

Figure 7. Heat map for pack animals microbial diversity at phylum level. The data were compared to M5RNA database using a maximum e-value of 1e–5, a minimum identity of 80% and a minimum alignment length of 50 bp.

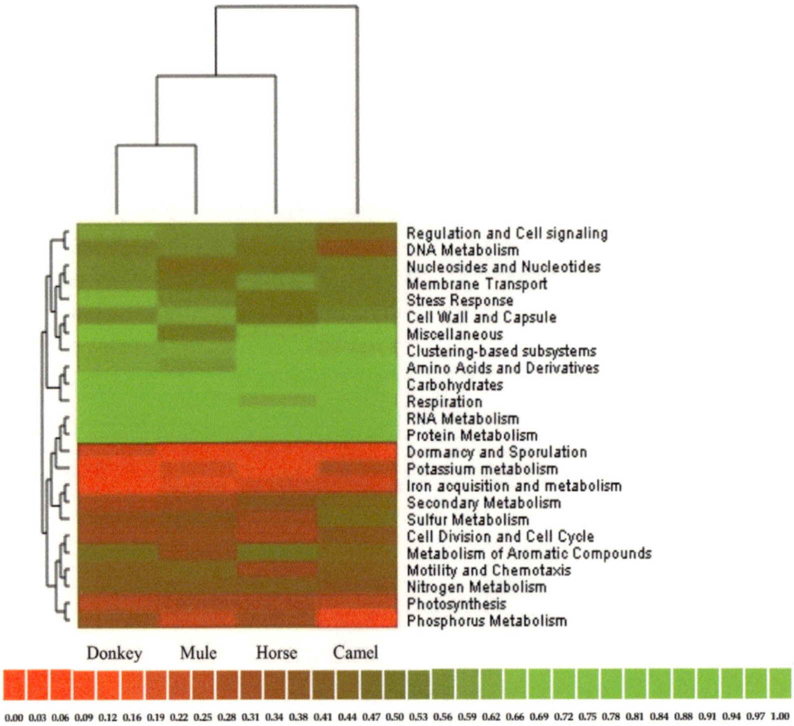

Figure 8. Heat map for pack animals microbial diversity at functional level. The data were compared to SEED subsystems using a maximum e-value of 1e–5, a minimum identity of 80% and a minimum alignment length of 30 measured in aa for protein.

Acknowledgements

The authors acknowledge the facilities provided by ICAR-NRCC, Bikaner, and Department of Biotechnology, AAU, as well as the financial assistance provided by the VTC-Rumen microbes.

Author details

Suchitra Sena Dande*, Niteen V. Patil and Chaitanya G. Joshi

*Address all correspondence to: dssena26@gmail.com

ICAR-Directorate of Poultry Research, Hyderabad, India

References

[1] Fenchel T, Finlay BJ. Ecology and evolution in anoxic worlds. Oxford Series in Ecology and Evolution. 1995. ISBN 019-854838-9 (H.b.) and 019-854837-0 (P.b.)

[2] Woese CR, Kandler O, Wheelis ML. Towards a natural system of organisms: Proposal for the domains Archaea, Bacteria and Eucarya. Proceedings of the National Academy of Sciences United States of America. 1990;**87**:4576-4579

[3] Curtis TP, Sloan WT. Prokaryotic diversity and its limits: Microbial community structure in nature and implications for microbial ecology. Current Opinion in Microbiology. 2004;**7**:221-226

[4] Nichols D. Cultivation gives context to microbial ecologist. FEMS Microbiology Ecology. 2007;**60**(3):351-357

[5] Staley JT, Konopka A. Measurement of in situ activities of nonphotosynthetic microorganisms in aquatic and terrestrial habitats. Annual Review in Microbiology. 1985;**39**:321-346

[6] Torsvik V, Ovreas L. Microbial diversity and function in soil: From genes to ecosystems. Current Opinion in Microbiology. 2002;**5**(3):240-245

[7] Riesenfeld CS, Schloss PD, Handelsman J. Metagenomics: Genomic analysis of microbial communities. Annual Review in Genetics. 2004;**38**:525-552

[8] Turnbaugh PJ, Ley RE, Hamady M, Fraser-Liggett CM, Knight R, Gordon JI. The human microbiome project. Nature. 2007;**449**:804-810

[9] Dinsdale EA, Edwards RA, Hall D, et al. Functional metagenomic profiling of nine biomes. Nature. 2008;**452**:629-632

[10] Frias-Lopez J, Shi Y, Tyson GW, Coleman ML, et al. Microbial community gene expression in ocean surface waters. Proceedings of the National Academy of Sciences United States of America. 2008;**105**:3805-3810

[11] Qu A, Brulc JM, Wilson MK, Law BF, et al. Comparative metagenomics reveals host specific metavirulomes and horizontal gene transfer elements in the chicken cecum microbiome. PLoS One. 2008;**3**:e2945

[12] Hess M, Sczyrba A, Egan R, Kim TW, et al. Metagenomic discovery of biomass-degrading genes and genomes from cow rumen. Science. 2011;**331**:463-467

[13] Ross EM, Moate PJ, Marett LC, Cocks BG, Hayes BJ. Metagenomic predictions: From microbiome to complex health and environmental phenotypes in humans and cattle. PLoS One. 2013;**8**(9):e73056. DOI: 10.1371/journal.pone.0073056.

[14] Pope PB, Mackenzie AK, Gregor I, Smith W, et al. Metagenomics of the Svalbard reindeer rumen microbiome reveals abundance of polysaccharide utilization loci. PLoS One. 2012;**7**:e38571

[15] Lamendella R, Jorge W, Santo Domingo, Shreya G, et al. Comparative fecal metagenomics unveils unique functional capacity of the swine gut. BMC Microbiology. 2011;**11**:103

[16] Swanson KS, Dowd SE, Suchodolski JE, Middelbos IS, et al. Phylogenetic and gene-centric metagenomics of the canine intestinal microbiome reveals similarities with humans and mice. ISME Journal. 2011;**5**(4):639-649

[17] Tringe SG, von Mering C, Kobayashi A, Salamov AA, et al. Comparative metagenomics of microbial communities. Science. 2005;**308**:554-557

[18] Dande SS, Bhatt VD, Patil NV, Joshi CG. The camel faecal metagenome under different systems of management: Phylogenetic and gene-centric approach. Livestock Science. 2015. DOI: http://dx.doi.org/10.1016/j.livsci.2015.05.024i

[19] Whiteley AS, Jenkins S, Waite I, Kresoje N, et al. Microbial 16S rRNA Ion Tag and community metagenome sequencing using the Ion Torrent (PGM) Platform. Journal of Microbiology Methods. 2012;**91**:80-88. DOI: 10.1016/j.mimet.2012.07.008

[20] Meyer F, Paarmann D, D'Souza M, Olson R, Glass EM, Kubal M. The metagenomics RAST server—A public resource for the automatic phylogenetic and functional analysis of metagenomes. BMC Bioinformatics. 2008;**9**:386

[21] EBI metagenomics—A new resource for the analysis and archiving of metagenomic data. Nucleic Acids Research. 1 January 2014;**42**(D1):D600-D606. DOI: 10.1093/nar/gkt961

[22] Mariat D, Firmesse O, Levenez F, Guimarães VD, et al. The Firmicutes/Bacteroidetes ratio of the human microbiota changes with age. BMC Microbiology. 2009;**9**:123. DOI: 10.1186/1471-2180-9-123

[23] Henrici AT, Johnson DE. Studies of freshwater bacteria. II. Stalked bacteria, a new order of Schizomycetes. Journal of Bacteriology. 1935;**30**:61-93

[24] Sakai T, Ishizuka K, Kato I. Isolation and characterization of a fucoidan-degrading marine bacterium. Marine Biotechnology. 2003;**5**:409-416

[25] Samsudin AA, Evans PN, Wright AD, Al Jassim R. Molecular diversity of the foregut bacteria community in the dromedary camel (*Camelus dromedarius*). Environmental Microbiology. 2011;**13**(11):3024-3035

[26] Bhatt VD, Dande SS, Patil NV, Joshi CG. Molecular analysis of the bacterial microbiome in the fore stomach fluid from the dromedary camel (*Camelus dromedarius*). Molecular Biology Reports. 2013. DOI: 10.1007/s11033-012-2411-2414

Chapter 6

Whole-Genome-Based Phylogeny and Taxonomy for Prokaryotes

Guanghong Zuo and Bailin Hao

Additional information is available at the end of the chapter

http://dx.doi.org/10.5772/intechopen.68563

Abstract

A faithful prokaryotic phylogeny should be inferred from genomic data and phylogeny determines taxonomy. The ever-growing amount of sequenced genomes makes this approach feasible and practical. Whole-genome phylogeny must be based on alignment-free methodology and should be verified by direct comparison with taxonomy at all ranks from domains down to species. When the number of genomes goes into tens of thousands, the realization of the above program also presents technical challenges. The power of a long-tested Web Server named Composition Vector Tree (CVTree) will be demonstrated on examples from mega-classification of bacteria to high resolution at and below the species level.

Keywords: alignment-free phylogeny, *Bacteria, Archaea*, CVTree, mega-classification, prokaryotic taxonomy

1. Introduction

Prokaryotes are the most successful creatures on Earth, comprising two of the three main domains of life [1, 2]: *Archaea* and *Bacteria*. It has been estimated that there are 10^{30} living cells [3] on the planet. Although the notion of prokaryotic species has been a subject of long debate, the estimated number of species, whatever the definition one adopts, surely exceeds 10^7 [4]. By contrast, for the time being only less than 14,000 species names have been validly published and come with a standing in nomenclature [5]. Nevertheless, though based on such rare sampling, bacterial phylogeny and systematics have made significant progress since the late 1970s mainly due to the use of 16S rRNA sequences as molecular markers [6, 7]. However, the fact that prokaryotic phylogeny becoming congruent with taxonomy on the basis of the same kind of markers calls for independent verification. The verification should preferably use different input data, for example, non-RNA sequences, and rely on distinct methodology, for example, an alignment-free approach. At present, convincing answers to the problem are naturally provided by making use of the ever-growing amount of genomic data.

In fact, the idea is by no means new. As early as in 1987, an "Ad Hoc" Committee on reconciliation of approaches to bacterial systematics stated in its report [8]:"There was general agreement that the complete deoxyribonucleic acid (DNA) sequence would be the reference standard to determine phylogeny and that phylogeny should determine taxonomy. Furthermore, nomenclature should agree with (and reflect) genomic information."

Furthermore, in the heyday of the human genome project Carl Woese stepped forward bravely with a manifesto for microbial genomics [9]. Woese wrote about the same time that "Genome sequencing has come of age, and genomics will become central to microbiology's future. It may appear at the moment that the human genome is the main focus and primary goal of genome sequencing but do not be deceived. The real justification in the long run is microbial genomics" [10].

The development of microbiology in subsequent years witnesses the foresight of Carl Woese. In particular, there has been continuing discussion on how to construct genome-based phylogeny and taxonomy, see, for example [11–14]. The abundance of genomic data enables the transition from comparing methodological suggestions to devising practical tools for bench microbiologists. In this chapter, we review our decade-long effort [15–20] to develop a whole-genome-based and alignment-free Composition Vector Tree (CVTree) approach and demonstrate the companion CVTree Web Server.

2. The CVTree approach

The CVTree approach is endowed with several distinctive features. It is based on whole genomes. It utilizes an alignment-free method for genome comparison. The resulting phylogenetic tree turns out to be essentially parameter free. The evaluation of the trees is realized by direct comparison with prokaryotic taxonomy. We elaborate these points in more detail in the subsequent text.

First of all, the feasibility of CVTree is guaranteed by the availability of the ever-growing amount of sequenced genomes. Since the first two bacterial genomes were published in 1995 [21, 22], the number of sequenced prokaryotic genomes has been accumulating rapidly. According to the GOLD Database [23], nearly 90,000 prokaryotic genomes have been deposited by the end of August 2016. The fact that more than half of the available genomes are incomplete or permanent drafts do not diminish the usefulness of these data, as nowadays annotation of genomic sequences may be easily carried out by using public-domain software or services such as IMG [24]. Moreover, the CVTree approach is insensitive to details of annotation. In principle, a whole genome contains most of phylogenetic information of an organism. Taking whole genomes as input data circumvents the selection of sequence segments or homologous proteins, thus eliminating ambiguity caused by human judgments. For example, lateral gene transfer, causing serious bias in phylogeny if based on a single or a few proteins, appears merely as a mechanism of genome evolution together with lineage-dependent gene loss.

http://dx.doi.org/10.5772/intechopen.68563

Second, prokaryotic genomes are extremely diverse in their size and gene content. For example, the five sequenced genomes of *Mycoplasma genitalium* have a median protein count of 484 and a genome size of 0.58 Mbp [22], whereas the largest bacterial genome sequenced so far, that of *Sorangium cellulosum* So0157-2 strain, consists of 10,174 proteins and 14.8 Mbp [25]. We did not mention the highly degenerated tiny genomes of some bacterial endosymbionts, which are not recommended to be included in a phylogenetic study of free-living organisms. More than 20-fold differences in protein number and genome size preclude comparison of these genomes by sequence alignments. In other words, a whole-genome-based prokaryotic phylogeny must be built by using alignment-free comparison of genomes.

Our way of being alignment-free consists in extending the notion of amino acid frequency ($K = 1$) to an alphabet made of 20^K oligo-peptides of length K ($K \geq 3$). By taking all the protein products encoded in a genome and counting the number of each type of the K-peptides by using a sliding window of width K, we construct a raw composition vector (CV) by arranging the counts in a lexicographical order of the K-peptides. A simple-minded way of using these CVs to represent species and defining species separation by the distance between CVs did not yield much meaningful results. Many researchers, along with the authors of this chapter, may have encountered this hurdle.

Upon reflection on Kimura's theory of neutral evolution [26], one realizes the necessity of subtracting a background caused by neutral mutations left in a genome. These neutral mutations have nothing to do with evolutionary process but contribute to components of the raw CVs. Since, according to Kimura, mutations occur randomly at molecular level, the neutral contributions to the K-peptide counts may be taken into account by invoking some statistical consideration as follows. First, collect the counts of all K-, (K-1)-, and (K-2)-peptides from the protein products of a genome. Then, predict the number of a given type of K-peptide from the counts of shorter ones by using a (K-2)-th Markov prediction [15, 16]. Suppose that for a certain type of K-peptide, the actual count coincides with the prediction. This would mean that the count of this particular K-peptide does not contain new phylogenetic information, as what added to the counts of (K-1)- and (K-2)-peptides is merely a statistical formula. What really matters is the difference between the actual count and the predicted number. Replacing each component of a raw CV by the corresponding difference, a "renormalized" CV is obtained. The subtraction procedure is crucial for success of the method, but we skip the mathematical details, as these can be found in previous publications, for example, in [15, 16] and [20]. We indicate that the key formula of the subtraction procedure may be derived in two independent ways, either by using the relation between joint probability and conditional probability [15, 16] or by applying the maximal entropy principle [27].

The peptide length K figuring in the above description looks like a parameter. However, it does not serve as a parameter since a fixed K is used for all genomes to generate a tree. The minimal value of $K = 3$ is dictated by the (K-2)-th Markov model itself. Larger K-values put emphasis on species specificity. The optimal value of K depends on the total amount of amino acids letters in all the protein sequences under study, $K = 5$ and 6 being the best for *Bacteria* and *Archaea*. For a detailed discussion on the role and choice of K, please consult [20].

Traditionally, the quality of phylogenetic trees is evaluated by statistical resampling procedures such as bootstrap or jackknife tests. However, successfully passing these tests tells at most the stability and self-consistency of the trees with respect to small variations in the input data, by far not the objective correctness of the branching scheme. We note that the CVTree results have passed both bootstrap and jackknife tests [28]. Furthermore, from the early CVTree constructed on 106 genomes [16] to trees based on 10,000 or more genomes, the agreement of CVTrees with taxonomy has kept improving. This fact may be taken as successfully passing larger and larger "anti-jackknife" tests. Therefore, we advocate the viewpoint that, instead of doing the time-consuming and indirect statistical resampling tests, the branching orders in a phylogenetic tree should be checked with the taxonomic hierarchy for the same set of input data. In fact, this is nothing but realization of the "general agreement" formulated in the 1987 Report of the Ad Hoc Committee [8].

A key notion in checking the agreement of phylogeny with taxonomy consists in monophyly. Introduced in 1866 by Ernst Huckael and originated from zoology, this notion requires the recognition of common ancestry, a requirement hardly satisfied by prokaryotes predominantly with asexual reproduction. Therefore, we take a pragmatic standpoint by restricting ourselves to the input dataset only. Being a reciprocal notion, monophyly applies to both taxonomy and phylogeny. An input data set comes with a reference taxonomy, in the case of CVTree, the NCBI taxonomy. If a taxon under study contains all the subordinate members inclusively, meaning that no member escapes to other taxon and no stranger from other taxon gets in, then the taxon is said to be monophyletic. Similarly, if a tree branch contains leaves representing species from one and the same taxon without strangers from other taxa, the branch is said to be monophyletic. In this sense, the genus *Clostridium* cannot be considered monophyletic in taxonomy, as many separate clusters are listed, including a big *senso stricto* group and many smaller clusters, see, for example, [29, 30]. Naturally, one cannot use the notion of monophyly to evaluate the *Clostridium* part of a tree. By the way, CVTree may help to bring the taxonomy of *Clostridium* to a better shape in the future.

3. The CVTree3 Web server

The underlying idea of CVTree and the corresponding algorithm described in the last section is simple in essence but hard to implement as many vectors and matrices of very high dimensions are involved. In order to help microbiologists to use this convenient tool, we have designed a public-domain Web Server called CVTree. The first CVTree Web Server was published in 2004 [31] and ceased service by now. An improved second release of 2009 [32] is still functioning [33]. However, we strongly recommend the users to try out the latest 2015 release CVTree3 [34] with many new functions added [35]. This is a much more powerful Web Server, which resides in a cluster with 64 cores and is capable to construct trees based on several thousands of genomes in a few minutes. In fact, all the descriptions in the subsequent sections refer to this latest version of Web Server.

Suffice it to type the above URL into the browser in order to enter the server without any login procedure. Leaving an email address is not obligatory but useful. As there is an online and printable help file, we skip most of the technicalities of how to use the server and concentrate on its characteristic features and typical results.

3.1. Input data set

The CVTree3 server is equipped with a built-in collection of genomes. For the time being, there are more than 3000 bacterial and archaeal genomes of a wide taxonomic assortment for picking up. These data are updated from time to time. Users can also upload their own genome data, 100 M compressed or not at a time. It is highly recommended to put the users' data on a wide taxonomic background no matter what kind of problem is studied. A background with broad sampling in taxonomy increases the stability of the results and allows outliers to escape to where they prefer. In order to avoid confusion, we mention in passing that many examples in this chapter are based on CVTrees built on 10,000 or more genomes.

3.2. Lineage information

Both built-in and user-uploaded genomes come with lineage information. For built-in genomes, the information is taken from the NCBI taxonomy [36] with minor corrections when necessary. Users should supply lineage information for the uploaded data. Lineage information for a genome looks like the following:

<D>Bacteria<K>Bacteria<P>Proteobacteria<C>Alphaproteobacteria<O>Caulobacterales<F> Caulobacteraceae<G>Caulobacter<S>Caulobacter_crescentus<T>Caulobacter_crescentus_ CB15_uid5789.NCBI

where <D>, <K>, <P>, <C>, <O>, <F>, <G>, <S>, and <T> stand for Domain, Kingdom, Phylum, Class, Order, Family, Genus, Species, and sTrain, respectively (for prokaryotes, <D> and <K> do not make difference; they are kept for future extension of CVTree to Eukarya). A missing or uncertain rank carries a fixed indicator "Unclassified", for example, <F>Unclassified denotes an as-yet-not-designated family.

We note that in the early days of whole-genome phylogenetic studies, say, in 2004 [16], genomes were given abbreviations in figures and tables. With the number of genomes growing into hundreds and thousands, it is more convenient for the experts to deal with fully fledged names including strain tags, and so on, as is done in CVTree3.

3.3. Interactive display of trees

Because it is hard to comprehend a phylogenetic tree with many thousands of leaves, CVTree3 is equipped with an interactive display capable of collapsing or expanding branches in the tree, keeping the overall topology unchanged. For example, when there are 179 genomes assigned to the class <C>*Epsilonproteobacteria* in the input data set and they all appear in a monophyletic branch, the whole branch may be collapsed into a single leaf labeled by the class name with the total number of genomes indicated in parentheses. In this way, the number of leaves in the whole tree may be greatly reduced, while the overall structure is clearly represented. In fact, at $K = 5$ or 6 a big CVTree usually appears in a maximally collapsed form with only three branches as shown in **Figure 1**.

In **Figure 1**, all three collapsed leaves would have appeared in red, because red color is used to represent monophyletic entries. If not monophyletic, they are usually shown in blue. Other

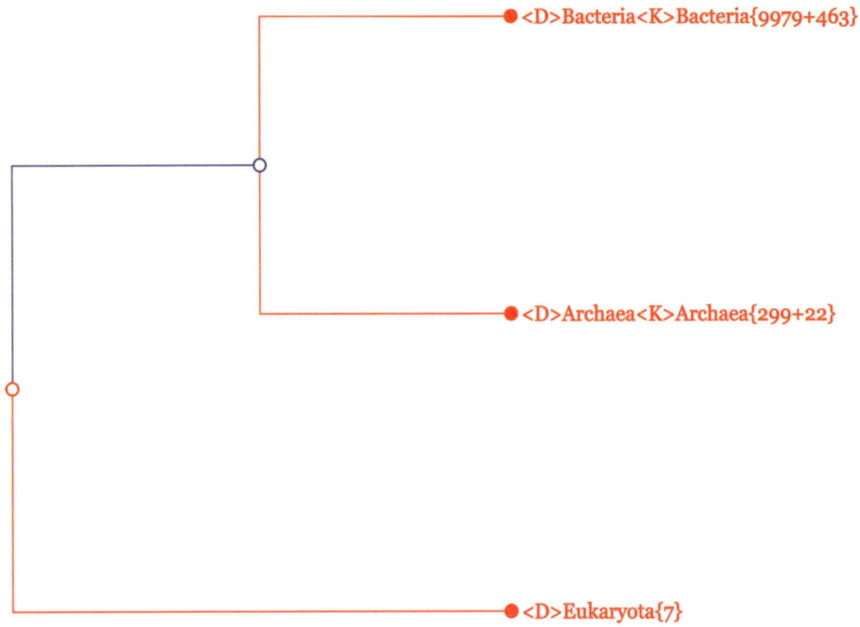

Figure 1. A maximally collapsed CVTree confirming the three main domains of life as suggested by Carl Woese. The numbers in the expression {9979+463} tell that there are 9979 genomes with complete lineage information and 463 with incomplete or absent information.

colors used in CVTree3 include green (taxon matching a Query) and purple (taxon with Unclassified rank). By the way, making an enquiry provides the quickest way to get to a taxon of interest. For example, typing *Epsilonproteobacteria* to replace "Query Search" in the preamble of the tree display immediately leads to a properly collapsed tree with the taxon in enquiry shown in green.

3.4. Lineage modification and re-collapsing a tree

A complete lineage may be incorrect. In some cases, an "unclassified" taxon name may be inferred from its neighborhood. When inspecting a tree, it may be tempting to modify some lineage information in order to reach better agreement between the tree-branching order and taxonomy. The CVTree3 Web Server provides a mechanism to demonstrate the consequences of trial lineage modifications. To this end, the user prepares a "Lineage Modification" file comprising separate lines of the following form:

old_lineage<space>new_lineage

(<space> means typing a space in between the two pieces of information). For example, there is a monophyletic genus *Aliivibrio* represented by eight genomes in CVTree. However, as a whole this cluster gets inserted into the genus *Vibrio* and thus violates the monophyly of the latter, as is shown in **Figure 2**.

Upon seeing this situation, one may wish to rename *Aliivibrio* simply as *Vibrio*. One adds the following line in the "Lineage Modification" file:

http://dx.doi.org/10.5772/intechopen.68563

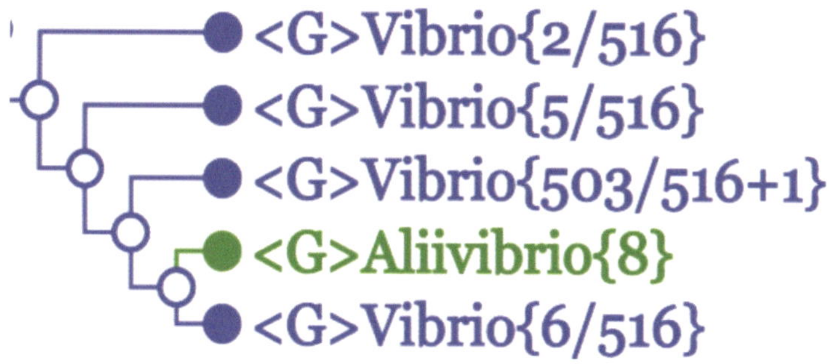

Figure 2. A monophyletic genus Allivibrio represented by eight genomes gets into the genus Vibrio and violates the monophyly of the latter. Vibrio{5/516} means this line represents five genomes out from a total of 516 Vibrio genomes.

<G>Aliivibrio <G>Vibrio

(sometimes more ranks must be included in order to make the modification unique) and then submit the file to the server for re-collapsing. After a while, a renewed tree appears in which the entries shown in **Figure 2** shrink to a single line <G>*Vibrio*{524}. Nevertheless, it must be emphasized that any actual lineage modification should be carried out in accordance with the International Code of Nomenclature of Prokaryotes [37] and be published in an appropriate journal. What described above only provides a trial means.

3.5. Report of taxa statistics

When comparing a tree containing thousands of leaves with an underlying taxonomy, one would like to check the overall "convergence," that is, how many taxa are monophyletic or non-monophyletic, at all taxonomic ranks from phyla down to species. The two previous releases of CVTree Web Server ran under a fixed peptide length K. It was up to the user to collect and observe the convergence of trees under different K. The CVTree3 Web Server, however, produces trees for several K-values in one run, say, for $K = 3$ to 9. This provides a new angle to evaluate the quality of the resulted trees. Obviously, it is not an easy job to accomplish if done manually. CVTree3 generates a summary table after each collapsing and re-collapsing. The summary is given as a long list arranged according to the taxonomic hierarchy. As a taxon that contains only a single species must be "embarrassingly" monophyletic, such items may be suppressed in the report. Take again the example given in the previous subsection. In the summary before doing the lineage modification, there is a monophyletic genus *Aliivibrio*{8} and a non-monophyletic genus *Vibrio*{516}. After making the modification only a monophyletic *Vibrio*{524} remains, but the total number of monophyletic genera does not change, as *Vibrio* adds to monophyletic ones but *Aliivibrio* drops out from the summary.

3.6. Output of print-quality sub-tree figures

Any part of a tree may be extracted to generate print-quality figures. The CVTree3 Web Server provides several formats for output. The formats include Encapsulated PostScript (.eps), Scalable Vector Graph (.svg), Portable Document File (.pdf), and Portable Network Graphics (.png). The output figures may be in the original colors or be made monochromatic.

4. Taxonomic resources for prokaryotes

Taxonomy has always been a work in progress. As we shall refer to taxon names and ranks repeatedly, it helps to indicate the main taxonomic resources used in our study.

4.1. The NCBI taxonomy database

The NCBI taxonomy database [36] carries a disclaimer after each entry that "it is not an authoritative source for nomenclature or classification." However, the NCBI taxonomy reflects much dynamic and up-to-date knowledge, as for any deposited molecule data, the authors would supply a piece of taxonomic information, not necessarily agreeing with the "generally accepted" opinion but better than none. This said, the NCBI taxonomy is taken as a start point for making a default Lineage Information file that comes with CVTree3.

4.2. Bergey's manual

The second edition of Bergey's Manual of Systematic Bacteriology [29], a grandiose work of more than 8600 pages, took 12 years (2001–2012) to accomplish. Upon its completion, Bergey's Manual Trust made it clear that this was the last hardcopy edition. Future editions would be electronic. In fact, the electronic Bergey's Manual of Systematics of Archaea and Bacteria, abbreviated as BMSAB, saw the light at the end of 2015 in the Wiley Online Library [30]. We note that BMSAB is organized on the basis of genera and many genus descriptions are taken from the previous volumes of Bergey's Manual [29] without any change.

4.3. The Prokaryotes IV

The Prokaryotes, a collective multivolume work, has its fourth edition [38] published in 2013–2014. Six volumes out of a total of 11 are devoted to classifications of *Bacteria* and *Archaea*. The taxa are divided basically by families with historical accounts as well as some emphasis on genera and species proposed after the corresponding volumes of Bergey's Manual [29]. Volumes in this fourth edition draw much information from the All-Species Living Tree project [39, 40] which is an initiative of the journal Systematics and Applied Microbiology in collaboration of a group of European microbiologists to reconstruct a single phylogenetic tree based on 16S rRNA sequences for all available type strains of *Bacteria* and *Archaea*. The latest release (*http://www.arb-silva.de/projects/living-tree/*) LTPs123 of September 2015 was based on 11,490 *Bacteria* and 449 *Archaea* sequences. In what follows, the All-Species Living Tree is abbreviated as LVTree when needed.

4.4. International Journal of Systematic and Evolutionary Microbiology

International Journal of Systematic and Evolutionary Microbiology (IJSEM) is the standard place to publish taxonomic proposals. Proposals published in a few journals other than IJSEM only make a small fraction of that in IJSEM. Taken altogether, about 800 new taxa appear yearly for the time being. As there is necessarily a time lag for new taxa to be recorded in BMSAB [30] or in The Prokaryotes IV [38], one must take into account data published in periodicals such as IJSEM and alike. To this end, a timely and helpful resource is the List of Prokaryotes with Standing in Nomenclature, abbreviated as LPSN [5]. Speaking about nomenclature, one must note that a preliminary draft of the long-due revision of International Code of Nomenclature of Prokaryotes (subtitled as 2008 Revision) has appeared in IJSEM in 2015 [37].

5. Applications of CVTree

Now, we are prepared to summarize the success of the CVTree approach and to discuss its prospective.

5.1. Retrospective verifications of CVTree

First of all, taxonomic revisions published in recent years all agree with the branching orders in CVTrees without exceptions as long as the corresponding sequenced genomes are available for comparison. In particular, 16 such cases were listed in [34]. This kind of agreements may be taken as retrospective verifications of CVTree results. A recent example deals with a debate on the taxonomic placement of *Eubacterium rectale* when CVTree results support the objection to reclassify this species into a new genus *Agathobacter* [41]. Moreover, CVTree predicts that the species under debate should belong to an existing genus *Roseburia*. We mention two more examples among many. First, earlier predictions of CVTree helped to transfer *Cellvibrio gilvus* from the originally assigned class *Gammaproteobacteria* to the genus *Cellulomonas* in phylum *Actinobacteria* [19]. Second, CVTree revealed the wrong taxonomic assignment of *Burkholderia* JV3 strain and suggested to bring it to the genus *Stenotrophomonas* [19].

5.2. Mega-classification of Bacteria and Archaea

Cavalier-Smith [42] coined the term mega-classification for taxonomic demarcation of the ranks order, class, and higher. Up to present time, the highest taxonomic rank recognized by the International Code of Nomenclature of Prokaryotes [37] is class. A proposal to include the rank phylum in the Code appeared only quite recently [43]. With many thousands of sequenced genomes available nowadays, CVTree may help to improve the mega-classifications in many aspects. Due to space limitation of this chapter, we only briefly touch on some facts at the phylum level.

For the time being, more than 400 *Archaea* genomes have been sequenced. They are well organized at ranks above class or even order [44]. For example, the phylum *Crenarchaeota* contains a single class *Thermoprotei*; the phylum *Euryarchaeota* consists of eight to nine classes; the phylum *Thaumarchaeota* proposed a few years ago is also supported by CVTree. A few newly proposed but not yet fully established archaeal phyla may require more genomic data to confirm.

As regarding the bacterial branch, in CVTrees constructed by using 10,442 *Bacteria* genomes, an overwhelming majority of phyla comes out monophyletic without making any lineage modification or only with minor modifications (Ref. [34] where the tree was based on fewer genomes). **Table 1** compares all phyla which are monophyletic in LVTree with their counterparts in CVTree.

Phylum	LVTree	CVTree
Acidobacteria	25	17/19+4, Note 1
Actinobacteria	2897	1705/1742+26, Note 2
Aquificae	28	21
Armatimonadetes	3	2
Bacteroidetes	1240	649/651+14, Note 3
Caldiserica	1	1
Chlamydiae	13	131
Chlorobi	11	12
Chloroflexi	23	17
Chrysiogenetes	4	2
Cyanobacteria	16	198
Deferribacteres	11	6
Deinococcus_Thermus	84	54
Dictyoglomi	2	4
Elusimicrobia	6	2
Fibrobacteres	4	2
Fusobacteria	39	49
Gemmatimonadetes	1	2
Ignavibacteriae	2	4
Lentisphaerae	4	1
Nitrospirae	7	7
Planktomycetes	23	19
Spirochaetes	93	104, 12, 9+38, Note 4
Synergistetes	23	18
Tenericutes	186	193/203+1, Note 5
Thermodesulfobacteres	8	10
Thermotogae	43	57
Verrucomicrobia	43	22

Note 1. <F>Holophagaceae joins <O>Myxococcales in the next branch.

Note 2. <C>Coriobacteriia escapes from the main cluster of <P>Actinobacteria.

Note 3. Two genera from <F>Chitinophagaceae escape from the main cluster of the latter, separated by <P>Chlorobi and <P>Ignavibacteriae.

Note 4. <P>Spirochaetes splits into three disjoint orders separated by other phyla. See discussion below.

Note 5. <G>Acholeplasma escapes from <P>Tenericutes.

Numerals indicate the number of 16S rRNA sequences or genomes in each phylum. For the meaning of $n + m$, please see the caption of **Figure 1**.

Table 1. A comparison of monophyletic bacteria phyla in LVTree and CVTree.

In order to make the comparison more effective, we have transplanted many of the CVTree3 features to a LVTree Viewer [45]. Users are advised to make Query Search on the same taxon name alternately in CVTree3 Web Server and LVTree Viewer.

In spite of the "overemphasis on rRNA similarity as a single arbitrary criterion of relatedness" [42], the agreement between CVTree and LVTree at the phylum level is remarkable in **Table 1**.

Due to space limitation, we will not elaborate the Notes in **Table 1** except for making a remark on Note 4. The phylum *Spirochaetes* splits into three disjoint monophyletic clusters corresponding to the orders *Spirochaetales*, *Brachyspirales*, and *Bdellovibrionales*, each essentially containing one family. This might be the largest discrepancy between CVTree and LVTree phylogenies besides the two phyla discussed in the subsequent text.

In fact, two "big" phyla were absent in **Table 1**: *Proteobacteria* and *Firmicutes*. The phylum *Proteobacteria*, represented by the largest number of genomes, splits basically into two disjoint clusters. Most of the taxonomic uncertainties concentrate in the phylum *Firmicutes*. In fact, in the last 20 years, many new phyla have been extracted from *Firmicutes*, including *Actinobacteria* and *Tenericutes*, and the process still continues. As an example, **Figure 3** shows how *Coprothermobacter* takes the position of an independent phylum in CVTree. It was labeled as an "established phylum" in a 2004 census [46] but still listed in BMSAB [30] and The Prokaryotes IV [38] as a genus within *Firmicutes* with proviso.

5.3. Taxonomic position of newly sequenced genomes without proper standing in nomenclature

As the cost of sequencing, a bacterial genome drops below the expenses of average phenotyping experiments, many biological studies now start from genome sequencing. However, a substantial part of newly sequenced genomes appears without validly published names and proper lineage information. The corresponding teams are not interested and sometimes not in a position with budget and manpower to fill up the gap in compliance with the International Code of Nomenclature of Prokaryotes. After extracting the interested information, the genomes were dumped as Permanent Drafts. According to GOLD [23], Permanent Drafts make the most rapidly growing part of genomic data. If the situation persists, as Barny Whitman warned, the microbiological "literature will be once again be full of names of uncertain meaning, and the difficult work of several generations of microbial systematists will be undone" [47].

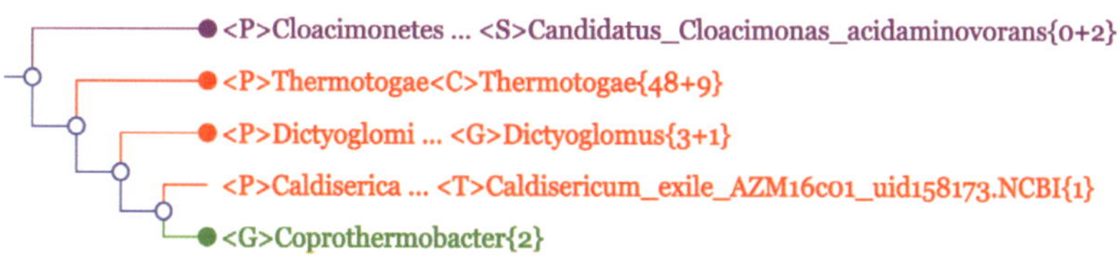

Figure 3. The genus *Coprothermobacter* from the phylum *Firmicutes* acquires status of a separate phylum. This figure also shows that Candidatus_Cloacimonas_acidaminovorans, an abundant bacterium in biogas reactors, actually takes the position of a phylum (formerly candidate phylum WWE1).

As an example, let us look at **Figure 4** which was cut from a CVTree based on 10,770 genomes. There is a genome with an illegal name Listeriaceae_bacterium_FSL_A5_0209. An inspection of its neighborhood hints on a plausible lineage like

<F>Listeriaceae<G>Listeria<S>Listeria_newyorkensis<T>Listeriaceae_bacterium_FSL_A5_0209

The line above assumes that it is a strain of an existing species, *L. newyorkensis*. Whether the assumption holds or not requires additional evidence by using other markers, a task often not possible or not worthwhile to do. In order to keep the possibility that this genome belongs to a new species other than *L. newyorkensis*, one may replace the <S> part of the lineage information by <S>Listeria_sp_FSL_A5_0209. This lineage modification eventually leads to a monophyletic genus *Listeria*{64} next to <G>*Brochothrix*{2}. The last two genera, taken together, make a monophyletic family *Listeriaceae*{66}. The two types of tags, "_sp_" and "_bacterium_," are frequently encountered in "illegal", that is, not validly published, names. As at the time of writing, in our genome warehouse, there are more than 6000 names that come with a tag "_bacterium_" and more than 2000 names that contain a tag "_sp_." These names may be at least partially improved by using CVTree, but not by LVTree as the latter excludes such names by design.

5.4. High resolution at the species level and below

Contrary to 16S rRNA sequence analysis, which does not possess high enough resolution at species and subspecies levels, CVTree approach distinguishes itself for extremely high-resolution power at infra-subspecific levels. This capability opens up new horizons in basic research as well as in applications. We briefly mention a few.

5.4.1. Population genetics of prokaryotes

Compared to Eukarya, the population genetics of prokaryotes is a much less studied subject. So far, only the clone structure of commensal *Escherichia coli* has been explored to some extent, see, for example, [48]. The major branches of *E. coli* strains in CVTree agree with the so-called phylogroups very well not only for the commensal groups A, B1, and B2 but also for pathogenic groups D and E, see Figure 5 in [34]. However, serotyping tests generate much finer divisions of *E. coli* strains and the correlation of serotypes with the branching orders in CVTrees has not been fully elucidated. In contrast to serotypes of *E. coli*, serotypes of *Streptococcus pyogenes* correlate well with CVTree branches [34].

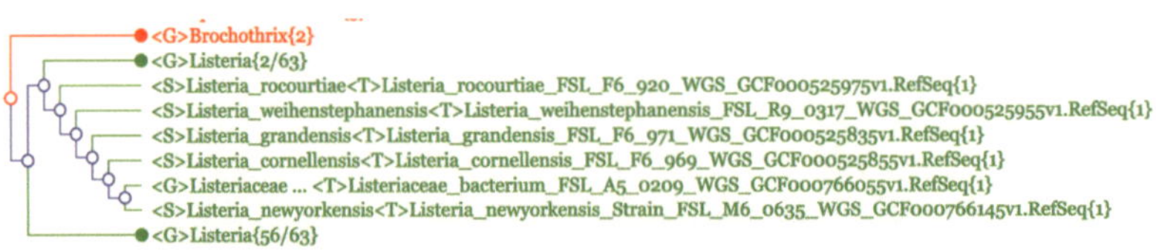

Figure 4. The questionable rank <G>*Listeriaceae* should be <G>*Listeria*; the illegal genome name Listeriaceae_bacterium_FSL_A5_0209 may be a new species Listeria_sp_FSL_A5_0209 requiring a formal name or a strain of the existing species Listeria_newyorkensis with strain tag FSL_A5_0209.

5.4.2. Distinguishing pathogenic bacteria species

Since the late 1980s, DNA-DNA hybridization (DDH) has become the standard measure to delineate bacteria species. As the clinically distinguishable *Yersinia pseudotuberculosis* and *Y. pestis* strains could not be resolved by using DDH, it was proposed to combine them into one and the same species. The proposal, however, was rejected by the Judicial Commission "because of possible danger to public health if there was confusion regarding *Y. pestis*, the plague bacillus" [49]. In CVTree, however, the corresponding strains go to different branches causing no problem in treating them as two species [19].

Another example concerns whether *Shigella* strains are clones within *E. coli* species or make individual species in the genus *Escherichia* on equal footing as *E. coli*. Even many sequence-based analyses put the former within the branches of the latter. Consequently, there seems to be a consensus that the genus name *Shigella* is kept only for historical and clinical reasons. CVTree's resolution again exceeds many other approaches by showing that the four well-described *Shigella* species are indeed sister species of *E. coli* within the same genus *Escherichia* [50].

5.4.3. Biogeography of bacteria

Geographic variations of multicellular plants and animals played an inspiring role for Charles Darwin to conceive the theory of evolution. Darwin did not mention microbes in his *Origin of Species* due to obvious limitations of his time. However, does it make sense to study geographic distribution of bacteria nowadays? The division of *Helicobacter pylori* into seven or more subpopulations carries geographic imprints which may be left by the migration of their human hosts [51]. The availability of more than 550 sequenced *H. pylori* genomes for the time being allows a much deeper study of the problem than a decade ago. A much more direct example without the intermediate influence of hosts is provided by "*Sulfolobus islandicus*" strains collected from various volcanic hot springs in Eurasian and North American continents. Genomic analyses including CVTree revealed that these clearly separated genomes should still be considered as geovars of the same species [52].

5.4.4. Electronic screening of bacterial strains

Many bacterial strains, naturally occurring in environment or intentionally made mutants, are screened for pathogenicity, drug-resistance, or metabolic products. These are costly and time-consuming jobs. When a certain amount of experimental data has been accumulated, mapping of the data onto a phylogenetic tree and picking up the most promising leaves for further exploration would significantly increase the efficiency of the screening process.

6. Concluding remarks

Biology starts from classification. However, the discipline of taxonomy is declining as less and less young scientists enter the field. The situation is especially true in microbiology. However, as eloquently pointed out by Barny Whitman, the supervisor of Bergey's Manual [29, 30], the solution lies in DNA sequencing and genomic analyses [47]. Recently, Whitman put forward a proposal to expand type material for naming prokaryotes to include DNA sequences [53]. With this proposal accepted by the microbiology research community, phylogeny and taxonomy of prokaryotes will ultimately become by-products of genomic analyses. Convenient and convincing phylogenomic tools such as CVTree are deemed to play an essential role in the future.

Acknowledgements

The work described in this chapter has been supported by the National Basic Research Program of China (973 Grant Nos. 2007CB814800 and 2013CB834100) and by the State Key Laboratory of Applied Surface Physics and Department of Physics of Fudan University.

Author details

Guanghong Zuo and Bailin Hao*

*Address all correspondence to: hao@mail.itp.ac.cn

T-Life Research Center and Department of Physics, Fudan University, Shanghai, China

References

[1] Woese CR, Fox GE. Phylogenetic structure of the prokaryotic domains: The primary kingdoms. Proceedings of the National Academy of Sciences United States of America. 1977;**74**:5088-5090

[2] Woese CR, Kandler O, Wheelis ML. Towards a natural system of organisms: Proposal for the domains of *Archaea, Bacteria,* and *Eucarya*. Proceedings of the National Academy of Sciences United States of America. 1990;**87**:4576-4579

[3] Whitman WB, Coleman DC, Wiebe WJ. Prokaryotes: The unseen majority. Proceedings of the National Academy of Sciences United States of America. 1998;**95**:6578-6583

[4] Editorial. Microbiology by numbers. Nature Reviews Microbiology. 2011;**9**:628. DOI:10.1038/nrmicro2644

[5] Parte AC. LPSN-list of prokaryotic names with standing in nomenclature. Nucleic Acids Research. 2014;**42:**D617-D616. DOI:10.1093/nar/gkt1111

[6] Fox GE, Pechman KR, Woese CR. Comparative cataloging of 16S ribosomal ribonucleic acid: Molecular approach to prokaryotic systematics. International Journal of Systematic Bacteriology. 1977;**27**:44-57

[7] Fox GE, Magrum LJ, Balch WE, Wolfe RS, Woese CR. Classification of methanogenic bacteria by 16S ribosomal RNA characterization. Proceedings of the National Academy of Sciences United States of America. 1977;**74**:4537-4541

[8] Wayne LG, Brenner DJ, Colwell RR, Grimont PAD, Kandler O, Krichevsky MI, Moore LH, Moore WEC, Murray RGE, Stackebrandt E, Starr MP, Truper HG. Report of the Ad Hoc Committee on reconciliation of approaches to bacterial systematics. International Journal of Systematic Bacteriology. 1987;**77**:463-464

[9] Woese CR. A manifesto for microbial genomes. Current Biology. 1998;**8**:R781-R783

[10] Woese CR. The quest for Darwin's grail. ASM News. 1999;**65**:260-263

[11] Coenye T, Gevers D, Van de Peer Y, et al. Towards a prokaryotic genomic taxonomy. FEMS Microbiology Reviews. 2005;**29**:147-167

[12] Konstantinidis KT, Tiedje JM. Prokaryotic taxonomy and phylogeny in the genomic era: Advancements and challenges ahead. Current Opinion in Microbiology. 2007;**10**:504-509

[13] Klenk H-P, Göker M. En route to a genome-based classification of *Archaea* and *Bacteria*?. Systematic and Applied Microbiology. 2010;**33**:175-182

[14] Chun J, Rainey FA. Integrating genomics into the taxonomy and systematics of the Bacteria and Archaea. International Journal of Systematic and Evolutionary Microbiology. 2014;**64**:316-324

[15] Hao B, Qi J, Wang B. Prokaryote phylogeny based on complete genomes without sequence alignment. Modern Physics Letters B. 2003;**17**:91-94

[16] Qi J, Wang B, Hao B. Whole proteome prokaryote phylogeny without sequence alignment: A K-string composition approach. Journal of Molecular Biology. 2004;**58**:1-11. DOI:10.1007/s00239-003-2493-7

[17] Gao L, Qi J, Sun J, Hao B. Prokaryote phylogeny meets taxonomy: An exhaustive comparison of composition vector trees with systematic bacteriology. Science in China Series C: Life Sciences. 2007;**50**:587-599. DOI:10.1007/s11427-007-0084-3

[18] Li Q, Xu Z, Hao B. Composition vector approach to whole-genome-based prokaryotic phylogeny: Success and foundations. Journal of Biotechnology. 2010;**149**:115-119. DOI:10.1016/j.jbiotec.2009.12.015

[19] Hao B. CVTrees support the Bergey's systematics and provide high resolution at species levels and below. The Bulletin of BISMiS. 2011;**2**:189-196

[20] Zuo G, Li Q, Hao B. On K-peptide length in composition vector phylogeny of prokaryotes. Computational Biology and Chemistry. 2014;**53**:166-173. DOI:10.1016/j.compbiolchem.2014.08.02

[21] Fleischmann RD, Adams MD, White O, Clayton RA, Kirkness EF, Kerlavage AR, et al. Whole-genome random sequencing and assembly of *Haemophilus influenzae* Rd. Science. 1995;**269**:496-512

[22] Fraser CM, Gocayne JD, White O, Adams MD, Clayton RA, Fleischmann RD, Bult CJ, Kerlavage AR, Sutton G, et al. The minimal gene complement of *Mycoplasma genitalium*. Science. 1995;**270**:397-404

[23] Reddy TBK, Thomas A, Stamatis D, Bertsch J, Isbandi M, Jansson J, Mallajosyula J, Pagani I, Lobos E, Kyrpides N. The genomes OnLine Database v.5:a metadata management system based on a four level (meta)genome project classification. Nucleic Acids Research. 2014;**43**:D1099-D1106. DOI:10.1093/nar/gku950

[24] Markowitz VM, Chen I-MA, Palaniappan K, Chu K, Szeto E, Pillay M, Ratner A, Huang J, Woyke T, Hutermann M, Anderson I, Billis K, Varghese N, Mavromatis K, Pati A, Ivanova NM, Kyrpies NC. IMG 4 version of the integrated microbial genomes comparative analysis system. Nucleic Acids Research. 2014;**42**:D560-D567. DOI:10.1093/nar/gkt963

[25] Han K, Li Z-F, Peng R, Zhu L-P, Zhou T, Wang L-G, Li S-G, Zhang X-B, Hu W, Wu Z-H, Qin N, Li Y-Z. Extraordinary expansion of a *Sorangium cellulosum* genome from an alkaline milieu. Scientific Reports. 2013;**3**:2101. DOI:10.1038/srep02101

[26] Kimura K. The Neutral Theory of Molecular Evolution. Cambridge University Press; 1984. p. 384

[27] Hu R, Wang B. Statistically significant strings are related to regulatory elements in the promoter region of *Saccharomyces cerevisiae*. Physica A. 2001;**290**:464-474

[28] Zuo G, Xu Z, Yu H, Hao B. Jackknife and bootstrap tests for the composition vector trees. Genomics Proteomics Bioinformatics. 2010;**8**:262-267. DOI:10.1016/S1672-0229(10) 60028-9

[29] Bergey's Manual Trust. Bergey's Manual of Systematic Bacteriology. 2nd ed. Vol. 1-5 New York, NY: Springer; 2001-2012. DOI:10.1007/b92997, 10.1007/978-0-387-68572-4, 10.1007/978-0-387-68233-4

[30] Whitman WB, et al., editors. Bergey's Manual of Systematics of Archaea and Bacteria. Online at John Wiley & Sons; 2015. DOI:10.1002/9781118960608

[31] Qi J, Luo H, Hao B. CVTree: A phylogenetic tree reconstruction tool based on whole genomes. Nucleic Acids Research. 2004;**32**:W45-W47. DOI:10.1093/nar/gkh362

[32] Xu Z, Hao B. CVTree update: A newly designed phylogenetic study platform using composition vectors and whole genomes. Nucleic Acids Research. 2009;**37**:W174-W178. DOI:10.1039/nar/gkp278

[33] CVTree Web Server [Internet]. 2009. Available from: http://tlife.fudan.edu.cn/cvtree [Accessed: 15-September-2016]

[34] Zuo G, Hao B. CVTree3 Web Server for whole-genome-based and alignment-free prokaryotic phylogeny and taxonomy. Genomics Proteomics Bioinformatics. 2015;**13**:321-331. DOI:10.1016/j.gpb.2015.08.004

[35] CVTree3 Web Server [Internet]. 2015. Available from: http://tlife.fudan.edu.cn/cvtree3 [Accessed: 15-September-2016]

[36] The NCBI Taxonomy Database [Internet]. 2016. Available from: https://www.ncbi.nlm.nih.gov/taxonomy [Accessed: 15-September-2016]

[37] Parker CT, Tindall BJ, Garrity GM, editors. International Code of Nomenclature of Prokaryotes. International Journal of Systematic and Evolutionary Microbiology. 2015;**1**:465-481. DOI:10.1099/ijsem.0.000778

[38] Rosenberg E, DeLong EF, Lory S, Stackebrandt E, Thompson F, editors. The Prokaryotes. 4th ed. Vol. 1-11 Berlin Heidelberg: Springer; 2013-2014. DOI:10.1007/978-3-642-31331-8, 10.1007/978-3-642-39044-9

[39] Yarza P, Richter M, Peplies J, Euzeby J, Amann R, Schleifer K-H, Ludwig W, Gloeckner FO, Rosselo-Mora R. The All-Species Living Tree project: A 16S rRNA-based phylogenetic tree of all sequenced type strains. Systematic and Applied Microbiology. 2008;**31**:241-250. DOI:10.1016/j.syapm.2008.07.001

[40] Yarza P, Sproer C, Swiderski J, Mrotzek N, Spring S, Tindall BJ, et al. Sequencing orphan species initiative (SOS): Filling the gaps in the 16S rRNA gene sequence database for all species with validly published names. Systematic and Applied Microbiology. 2013;**36**:69-73. DOI:10.1016/j.syapm.2012.12.006

[41] Zuo G, Hao B. Whole-genome-based phylogeny supports the objections against the reclassification of *Eubacterium rectale* to *Agathobacter rectalis*. International Journal of Systematic and Evolutionary Microbiology. 2016;**66**(6):2451. DOI:10.1099/ijsem.0.001407

[42] Cavalier-Smith T. The neomuran origin of archaebacteria, the negibacterial root of the universal tree and bacterial megaclassification. International Journal of Systematic and Evolutionary Microbiology. 2002;**52**:7-76

[43] Oren A, da Costa MS, Garrity GM, Rainey FA, Rosselo-Mora R, Schick B, Sutcliffe I, Trujilo ME, Whitman WB. Proposal to include the rank of phylum in the International Code of Nomenclature of Prokaryotes. International Journal of Systematic and Evolutionary Microbiology. 2015;**65**:4284-4287

[44] Zuo G, Xu Z, Hao B. Phylogeny and taxonomy of *Archaea*: A comparison of the whole-genome-based CVTree approach with 16S rRNA sequence analysis. Life. 2015;**5**:949-968. DOI: 10.3390/life5010949

[45] Zuo G, Zhi X, Xu Z, Hao B. LVTree Viewer: An interactive display for the all-species living tree incorporating automatic comparison with prokaryotic systematics. Genomics Proteomics Bioinformatics. 2016;**14**:94-102. DOI:10.1016/j.gpb.2015.12.002

[46] Schloss PD, Handeldsman J. Status of the microbial census. Microbiology and Molecular Biology Reviews. 2004;68:686-691. DOI: 10.1128/MMBR.68.4.686-691.2004

[47] Whitman WB. Intent of the nomenclatural code and recommendations about naming new species based on genomic sequences. The Bulletin of BISMiS. 2011;**2**:135-139

[48] Tenaillon O, Skurnik D, Picard B, Demamur E. The population genetics of commensal Escherichia coli. Nature Reviews Microbiology. 2010;8:207-217. DOI:10.1038/nrmicro2298

[49] Brenner DJ, Staley JT, Krieg NR. Classification of Prokaryotic Organisms and the Concept of Bacterial Speciation. Chapter 5 in Bergey's Manual [29]. Vol. 2B; 2002. pp. 27-32

[50] Zuo G, Xu Z, Hao B. *Shigella* strains are not clones of *Escherichia coli* but sister species in the genus *Escherichia*. Genomics Proteomics Bioinformatics. 2013;**11**:61-65. DOI: 10.1016/j.gpb.2012.11.002

[51] Falush D, Wirth T, Linz B, Pritchard JK, Stephens M, Kid M, et al. Traces of human migrations in *Helicobacter pylori* populations. Science. 2003;**299**:1582-1585

[52] Zuo G, Hao B, Staley JT. Geographic divergence of "*Sulfolobus islandicus*" strains assessed by genomic analyses including electronic DNA hybridization confirms they are geovars. Antonie van Leeuwenhoek. 2014;**105**:431-435. DOI: 10.1007/s10482-013-0081-4

[53] Whitman WB. Modest proposals to expand the type material for naming of prokaryotes. International Journal of Systematic and Evolutionary Microbiology. 2016;**66**:2108-2112. DOI: 10.1099/ijsem.0.000980